W0106220

CHILDREN
WITH CANCER
Mainstreaming and Reintegration

Edited by

Jan van Eys, M.D., Ph.D.
Department of Pediatrics
The University of Texas System
   Cancer Center
M.D. Anderson Hospital and
   Tumor Institute
Houston, Texas

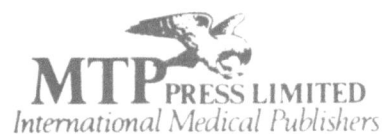
MTP PRESS LIMITED
International Medical Publishers

Published in the UK and Europe by
MTP Press Limited
Falcon House
Lancaster, England

Published in the US by
SPECTRUM PUBLICATIONS, INC.
175-20 Wexford Terrace
Jamaica, N.Y. 11432

Copyright © 1982 Spectrum Publications, Inc.

Softcover reprint of the hardcover 1st edition 1982

All rights reserved. No part of this book may be reproduced in any form, by
photostat, microform, retrieval system, or any other means without prior
written permission of the copyright holder or his licensee.

ISBN-13: 978-94-011-6700-0   e-ISBN-13: 978-94-011-6698-0
DOI: 10.1007/978-94-011-6698-0

Contributors

William G. Bartholome, M.D.
Department of Pediatrics, The
University of Texas Health Science
Center at Houston, Medical School

Dayle Bebee, L.L.D., Attorney
Austin, Texas

Dennis L. Coburn
Woodlands, Texas

Donna R. Copeland, Ph.D.
Department of Pediatrics, The
University of Texas System
Cancer Center

Elizabeth Deuble
Principal, Sinclair Elementary
School, Houston, Texas

Albert E. Gunn, M.B.,B.Ch.,L.L.B.
Medical Director, Rehabilitation
Center, The University of Texas
System Cancer Center

Paul Hansen
Area V, Executive Director for
Special Education, Houston
Independent School District

Rose Hicks
Associate Superintendent for
Special Education, Houston
Independent School District

Tom A. Holland, Ph.D.
Area I, School Psychologist
Houston Independent School
District

Charles A. LeMaistre, M.D.
President, The University of Texas
System Cancer Center

Katy Maxwell, Ph.D.
Grady School, School Psychologist
Houston Independent School
District

Sue Ann Nichols, R.N.
Head Nurse, Pediatric Clinic
Houston, Texas

Betty Pfefferbaum, M.D.
Department of Psychiatry, The
University of Texas Health Science
Center at Houston, Medical School

Billy Reagan
Superintendent, Houston
Independent School District

Charles R. Shaw, M.D.
Professor of Biology
Associate Professor of Psychiatry
Department of Pediatrics &
Biology, The University of Texas

Patricia M. Shell
Deputy Superintendent for Special
Services, Houston Independent
School District

Allison M. Stovall, M.S.W.
Department of Social Services
Department of Pediatrics
The University of Texas System
Cancer Center, M. D. Anderson
Hospital and Tumor Institute

Virginia Thompson, R.N., M.Ed.,
M.P.H., Executive Director of
School Health Services, Houston
Independent School District

Catherine van Eys, M.A.
Regional Day School Program for
the Deaf, Houston Independent
School District

Jan van Eys, M.D., Ph.D.,
Head, Department of Pediatrics,
The University of Texas System
Cancer Center

Mrs. Judy Warco, Parent

Mr. Jim Wright, Parent

Preface

Probably no two topics have generated more workshops, conferences, and lectures in medicine and education than the chronically ill child and the mandate of Public Law 94-142. In spite of the numerous examinations of these topics there has never been a serious dialogue between medical professionals and educators with the child as the focus. These proceedings represent such a unique event. The paradigm of the medically exceptional child is the child with cancer, a child with a life-threatening illness, but also a child with a high probability of being cured of this acute disease. Such a cure is purchased at a cost of late sequelae of disease and treatment alike. There is prejudice against this child. There is overt physical exceptionality. Therefore, the Fifth Annual Mental Health Conference of The University of Texas System Cancer Center, Department of Pediatrics, was a stimulus to generate this dialogue. When two nationally recognized giants in their respective fields, The University of Texas System Cancer Center and the Houston Independent School District, address a problem, the result transcends local concern. This conference goes far beyond the problem of the child with cancer to deal with all medically exceptional children. The focus on the needs and expectations for the child makes this workshop universal in application.

Education and medical care have only one common goal: healthy children who physically are optimally functional within the limitations imposed by nature and who mentally are able to cope with themselves as well as with the world. It is the coping with themselves that is the common goal presenting the greatest challenge. These proceedings show concepts that make it possible to attempt this task.

We the participants in this conference hope that our flashes of insight can be shared by professionals in medicine and education, and parents alike. The focus of this conference was the child, not how to comply with the law nor how to impose the authority of medicine on a child's life. Therefore, these proceedings are unique in the dialogue among educators, health care professionals, and parents, and in the concern for the child, which will help all adults, responsible for understanding and helping the medically exceptional child.

Jan van Eys

Acknowledgments

The Fifth Annual Mental Health Conference was an exciting venture between the school and the cancer center, just at a time when our government in its wisdom separated medicine and education. All those who worked so hard at maintaining a joint approach to the child through this conference deserve praise and thanks. A special word of gratitude must be reserved for Mr. John Carter Brooks who patiently edited the manuscripts. Without his assistance, the workshop publication would not have become a reality.

Contents

Workshop Introduction for The University of Texas System Cancer Center

CHARLES A. LeMAISTRE

It is a pleasure to introduce the Fifth Annual Mental Health Conference presented by the Department of Pediatrics at The University of Texas System Cancer Center. This meeting is particularly significant because it is cosponsored this year by the Houston Independent School District.

The joint sponsorship of the mental health conference is evidence of the very important subject matter to be discussed. As a result of greatly improved treatment for many forms of childhood cancer, more children than ever before are able to resume normal lives and return to school. Children with cancer need school. It is where they find the companionship of their contemporaries. And school offers a natural way to bring the child's life back to normal.

There have been major advances in the control and cure of childhood cancers. But, as in many fields, success often uncovers other problems. With longer life spans, we now see that work with these children does not end when they are cured or the cancer is controlled. Our support must continue until each child is fully integrated into the family, into society, and into school.

The successful reintegration of the child into his or her social milieu is as important as the successful management of the disease. Children have specific and unique problems. We still have very

1

little genuine understanding of the problems a child who has cancer faces. Until recently, these problems were not a chief concern because the outlook for children with cancer was not as good as it is today.

That the Houston Independent School District has been willing to cosponsor this meeting is characteristic of the attention given to the exceptional child. The District's interest in this topic demonstrates a sincere desire to meet a developing need and to prepare techniques that will truly reintegrate a child with cancer into the mainstream of the educational system.

The program will give a unique opportunity for conversation among many concerned people of different disciplines. I trust that the meeting will serve as the genesis for many programs that will aid the child with cancer.

Workshop Introduction for The Houston Independent School District

BILLY REAGAN

For the Houston Independent School District to be a part of this conference is seen as a distinct honor and privilege, for M.D. Anderson Hospital represents the highest dedication and service to mankind through its leadership in dealing with one of our most serious maladies.

Our whole thought and attitude about the outlook for the child with cancer has had to undergo a significant change. The possibility that the child with cancer is indeed cured, albeit at a price, forces us to incorporate this very special child into the mainstream of our education.

The Houston Independent School District has placed a great deal of effort and emphasis on the program of Magnet Schools in order to meet the needs of special students and student groups. This program has been extremely successful. It has changed the attitude towards the concern of special groups to meeting the need of each child in their specific way.

A new concern, and a new special group of children, must now be added to this planning. With the Houston Independent School District and M.D. Anderson Hospital together there is an opportunity to serve these children, both by continuing a program of education when the child is undergoing treatment in the hospital and by helping the child to be reintegrated into the school environment after hospitalization is completed. I am confident that our hospital and school personnel working together for the reintegration of medically exceptional children can bring about quantum jumps in education treatment for these children that have already been made in their medical treatment.

In addition, the strides made in the treatment of cancer and the consequent challenge to the educational system is but a paradigm for all chronic illnesses in childhood. The participants in this conference therefore have a general responsibility to formulate the insights and translate the visions into programs that will optimize the outcome for the very special child that the child with cancer represents.

Section I

SETTING THE TONE

CHAPTER 1

Reintegration of the Medically Exceptional Child

JAN VAN EYS

The reintegration of the medically exceptional child is a classic problem of defining what the clear need of the individual child is and how a system can be changed so that all individual problems are routinely solved. One can handle the occasional exceptional child on an ad hoc basis. But the overall problem of the medically exceptional child is enormous (Table 1) (1). The individual need, however, is the dominant force that makes for change. Cancer in children is a useful model because it illustrates so clearly the forces at work at the individual level that shape the response of the system as a whole. There is a major problem of reintegration of the medically exceptional child, as the following newspaper clipping will attest. It is reproduced in its entirety from the *Houston Chronicle* of February 27, 1980, under the headline: Misunderstanding. Cancer victim's wig causes fuss.

> Mesquite, Texas (AP) — North Mesquite High School Principal John Campbell says a confrontation with a cancer patient wearing a wig who was told his hair was too long was all a misunderstanding.
>
> But the teen-ager's mother said Tuesday the incident was inexcusable.
>
> The teen-ager, who suffers from bone cancer, lost his hair as a side effect of chemotherapy treatments and said he has worn the same wig to school since last April.
>
> The School district has cracked down on the hair rule since

**Table 1. Estimated Number of Exceptional Children
Served* and Unserved by Type of Exceptionality**

			TOTAL CHILDREN SERVED AND UNSERVED** (1974–1975)	PER CENT SERVED
TOTAL				
	AGE	0–19	7,886,000	50
	AGE	6–19	6,699,000	55
	AGE	0–5	1,187,000	22

From American Academy of Pediatrics (1).

*Estimated total numbers of medically exceptional children served—obtained from state education agency's (SEA) fall and winter 1978. Information by type of exceptionality was projected by SEA's for school year 1972–1973.

**Total number of medically exceptional children ages 0 to 19 provided on basis of estimates from various sources, including national agencies and organizations and state and local directories of special education. According to these sources, the incidence levels by types of medical exceptionality are as follows: speech impaired 3.5%, mentally retarded 2.3%, learning disabled 3.0%, emotionally disturbed 2.0%, crippled and other health impaired 0.5%, deaf 0.08%, hard of hearing 0.5%, visually handicapped 0.1%, deaf-blind and other multiply handicapped 0.06%. The total number of exceptional children in the above categories represents 12.035% of all school age children from 6 to 19 and 6.018% of all children 0 to 5 years. The population figures to which the incidence rates were applied were obtained from the Bureau of Census and reflect the population as of July 1, 1974.

the code was challenged by a student in court earlier this month and a state district judge ruled the school district could set and enforce its own dress and grooming standards for students.

But Campbell said, "No student has ever been disrespected in any manner in the 11 years I have been principal here. If something was said to that young man about a wig that was not groomed, I assure you no one knew it was a wig."

Ganze, who lost his left leg to cancer a year ago, said his collar-length wig was approved by school officials earlier in the year.

Campbell also denied reports from students that 150 boys in the 2,600-student high school were expelled Friday because of long hair.

The special needs of the child with cancer were not heeded. Clearly, one concern of school management overshadowed another.

The magnitude of the problem of childhood cancer is growing because children with cancer may now live indefinitely. The cure rate of cancer in children is well over the fifty percent mark. The problem is no longer confined to adjusting to a child who will die. That was until recently the tone of the medical-educational dialogue (2,3), if any existed at all. Cure brings an entirely different perspective to the educational prospect for the child. The school does need to accommodate the child, and the school is more than a matter of factual education. It is also an arena for socialization of the child. The concepts of society are introduced and taught in the schools. Many argue that the task of schools is nevertheless only teaching facts, and that the schools have no concern with the child's bodily health, except in so far that it must be possible for all children to partake of the education. However, that is clearly not the official concept. Miller, while discussing the legal basis of schools and health concerns in Indiana, quotes a ruling of a Minnesota Court, handed down as early as 1910 (4):

(The) education of a child means much more than merely communication to it the content of textbooks. . . . The physical and medical powers of the individual are so interdependent that no system of education, though designed solely to develop mentality, would be complete which ignored bodily health.

Schooling, even at its most conservatively purist, cannot ignore the whole being of a child. A child with cancer is a child who is normal in spite of the cancer and for whom having cancer is precisely being normal (5). The experience of having cancer molds those children into the individuals they are. They could not be anybody else. Without having had cancer they would never be the individuals they now are. Curing the cancer does not erase the experience, but allows the life to go on. For schools the question has been raised: "Can the child be distracted from his disease?" and the answer clearly is: "Of course not, but neither can we!" (6).

There are many concerns expressed regarding medical duties that might be placed on the teacher of the medically exceptional child (7). There is no doubt that such children may need medicines administered, that the schools may have to provide special diets, and that physical therapy needs to be actively pursued even when in school. Such concerns are not totally addressed by saying that teachers act *in loco parentis*. The teacher is a full member of the medical team.

The first and foremost need for solution of these near overwhelming problems is an understanding of the goals and needs for the child who is medically exceptional. We ought to understand and stipulate that schools have an effect on the eventual outcome and performance of the child (8). They are not just mechanical transmitters of knowledge. Therefore, the challenge to the schools is far greater than just removing physical barriers toward participation. Unfortunately, the model of care for the child with cancer, and in general the model of care for any child with a chronic medical affliction, is a medical one. The medical team is thought to need to teach all, but that model is not tenable. First of all, even if it were, the medical training is woefully lacking in preparing pediatric trainees to give guidance in the care of the medically exceptional child. A recent symposium drew attention to the problem and suggested avenues for remedy (9). However, that is not enough because it does not challenge the model. The education in school and the medical care must be part of a total package of professional support of child and family in preparing the child for a meaningful, productive, and self-confident life. School and medical care are not necessarily equal partners. Which predominates depends entirely on the need of the individual child. It is true that medical problems may overwhelm social concerns. To ignore the medical needs of a child with cancer will usually cause the child to die. On the other hand, following the medical regimen faithfully may result in cure in over fifty percent of all children. But precisely because of that change in outlook, we must deal with the total needs of the child (10). The medical establishment itself needs to be broadened. At M. D. Anderson Hospital, we divided the care in three conceptual sets: the cure by physicians, the care by nurses, and the adaptation to the disease by mental health workers. However, that is still not sufficient: society demands as goal an independent function for the child. Society insists that children acquire a norm of behavior, a set of common values, and a minimal body of skills and knowledge. That goal is much more formidable in scope than the medical task of making it possible to begin to participate in society. The two are so intertwined that they are neither separable nor sequential. It is possible to prepare the child for the future while medical care is still ongoing and even when the outcome is yet in doubt. It has been demonstrated that the most dreary aspects of medical care, the deadly hours in a waiting room, can be made a constructive part of the total care (11). How much more ought it to be possible to generate positive educational experiences while the cancer care is still ongoing? Two experienced teachers have, in fact, reported that it is quite achievable (12,13).

Therefore, professionals in education and medicine must work together. They must have mutual respect through understanding. This conference is a serious attempt at initiating meaningful dialogue and mutual instruction. The participants and the audience were drawn from the Houston Independent School District and the Department of Pediatrics of The University of Texas System Cancer Center. The problems these institutions encounter are representative of all urban school districts and comprehensive cancer centers. The problems these two institutions must devise solutions for are fully representative of the challenges of meeting the needs through the services of a large system. The speakers and discussors here are experts who must solve these problems daily: administrators who are frustrated because their staff hide behind the system; care givers who feel their administration is insensitive to the special needs of their one specific charge; parents who feel both lag behind in delivering the special help their children are perceived to need.

There is a need for effective communication to successfully reintegrate the child with cancer, as with any medically exceptional child, back into society. Cyphert has suggested the simple matrix of *who* needs to know against *what* needs to be known (14). The sets who need to know are the child, the medical team, the educational team, the family, and the fellow students. What they need to know falls into the subsets of knowledge, skills, and attitudes. Of these, attitudes are ultimately the most important (8). Even in medicine, not expecting cure can readily generate self-fulfilling prophesies (15). That phenomenon is well described in education, and occurs no less in medicine. To change attitudes, the teacher and the doctor must feel secure in their skills. That is the responsibility of each group of professionals, though through conferences such as these, they should sharpen those skills through outside critique. To be able to design skills the teacher should have knowledge. There are precious few data on the problems encountered by the child with cancer on return to the classroom. There are a number of papers at the "feeling" level, but factual descriptions and tabulations are few. Fortunately, data are beginning to emerge (16–20). That problems do exist ought to have been known. School phobia is far more prominent among children with cancer than among the general population (21).

It is not useful to have to painfully relearn experiences that others have learned. Their insights can be transmitted and assimilated. Therefore, this book is published so that educators and health care professionals understand that communication and cooperation are possible. In that process a certain ritualization of approach might occur that would not at all be bad. Walter Lippman once said, speaking of the world at large (22):

The real environment is altogether too big, too complex, and too fleeting for direct acquaintance. And although we have to act in the environment, we have to reconstruct it on a simpler model before we can manage with it. The analyst of public opinion must begin then, by recognizing the triangular relationship between the scene of action, the human picture of that scene, and the human response to that picture working itself out upon the scene of action.

This book attempts to do just that for the microcosm of the education of the handicapped. The medically exceptional child is, in fact, officially recognized as a child with a hidden handicap (23). The advent of Public Law 94-142 has perturbed the system as it was. This current sociological experiment makes it not only opportune to see the impact of this needed new cooperation between education and medicine, but makes it feasible to efficiently challenge past behavior and belief. Therefore, much of the discussion that follows centers around the meaning, impact, and consequences of that law. However, the conference deals primarily with the individual child forced to seek care *and* education in large systems with wide ranging input into standards of care and management. This conference deals with what is "best" for a particular child, but concludes as others have noted (24) that this is an indeterminate standard. Experiences were shared, concepts defined and explained, and a usable, simple model was constructed, out of which the care giver and educator of the future can construct a working model for each particular child entrusted to care.

FOOTNOTES

(1) The relevance of this quote was shown in the book by Erik Erikson: Toys and Reasons. Stages in the Ritualization of Experience. New York: W.W. Norton and Company, Inc., 1977. Erikson uses the quote himself (page 27).

REFERENCES

1. Committee on School Health, American Academy of Pediatrics. School Health: A Guide for Health Professionals. Evanston, Ill.: American Academy of Pediatrics, 1977.
2. Greene, P. The child with leukemia in the classroom. Am. J. Nurs., 75: 86–87, 1975.
3. Kaplan, D. M., Smith, A., Grzobstein, R. School management of the seriously ill child. J. Sch. Health, 44:250–254, 1974.
4. Miller, D. F. Legal bases for health practices in Indiana. J. Sch. Health, 40:446–450, 1970.
5. van Eys, J. The normally sick child. In: van Eys, J., ed. The Normally Sick Child. Baltimore: University Park Press, 1979, pp. 11–27.
6. Issner, N. Can the child be distracted from his disease? J. Sch. Health, 43:469–471, 1973.
7. Trahms, C. M., Afleck, J. Q., Lowenbraun, S., Scranton, T. A. The special educator's role on the health service team. Except. Child., 43: 344–349, 1977.
8. Rutter, M. School influences on children's behavior and development. (The 1979 Kenneth Blackfin Lecture, Children's Hospital Medical Center, Boston.) Pediatrics, 65:208–220, 1980.
9. Guralnick, M. J., Richardson, H. B., Jr. Pediatric Education and the Needs of Exceptional Children. Baltimore: University Park Press, 1980.
10. van Eys, J. The outlook for the child with cancer. J. Sch. Health, 47: 165–169, 1977.
11. Hoffman, J., Futterman, E. H. Coping with waiting. Psychiatric intervention and study in the waiting room of a pediatric oncology clinic. Compr. Psychiatry, 12:67–81, 1971.
12. Kirten, C., Liverman, M. Special educational needs of the child with cancer. J. Sch. Health, 47:170–173, 1977.
13. Kalinowski, S. Learning in adversity. In: van Eys, J., ed. The Normally Sick Child. Baltimore: University Park Press, 1979, pp. 39–44.
14. Cyphert, F. R. Back to school for the child with cancer. J. Sch. Health, 43:215–217, 1973.
15. van Eys, J. The truly cured child—The realistic and necessary goal in pediatric oncology. In: Spinetta, J. J., Deasy-Spinetta, P., eds. Living with Childhood Cancer. (Proceedings of a workshop, February, 1–3, 1980, San Diego, Calif.) St. Louis: C. V. Mosby Co., 1981, pp. 30–40.
16. Holmes, H. A., Holmes, F. F. After ten years, what are the handicaps and life styles of children treated for cancer? Clin. Pediatr., 14:819–823, 1975.

17. Zwartjes, W. J. Education of the child with cancer. American Cancer Society Proceedings of the National Conference on the Care of the Child with Cancer, 1979, pp. 150–155.

18. Zwartjes, W. J. The psychological cost of cure in the child with cancer. In: van Eys, J., Sullivan, M. P., eds. Status of the Curability of Childhood Cancers. (24th Annual Clinical Conference, M. D. Anderson Hospital and Tumor Institute, Houston) New York: Raven Press, 1980, pp. 277–284.

19. Deasy-Spinetta, P., Spinetta, J. J. The child with cancer in school; teacher's appraisal. J. Pediatr. Hematol–Oncol., 2:89–94, 1980.

20. Deasy-Spinetta, P. The school and the child with cancer. In: Spinetta, J. J., Deasy-Spinetta, P., eds. Living with Childhood Cancer. (Proceedings of a workshop, February 1–3, 1980, San Diego, Calif.) St. Louis: C. V. Mosby Co., 1981, pp. 153–168.

21. Lansky, S. B., Lowman, J. T., Vats, T., Gyulay, J. School phobia in children with malignant neoplasms. Am. J. Dis. Child, 129:42–46, 1975.

22. Lippman, W. Public Opinion. New York: Macmillan, Inc., 1960, pp. 15–16.

23. The White House Conference on Handicapped Individuals, Volume II. Final Report, Part C. Washington, D.C.: U.S. Government Printing Office, 1977, p. 283.

24. Mnookin, R. H. Children's rights. Legal and ethical dilemmas. The Pharos, 41:2–7, 1978.

CHAPTER 2

Good Intentions Become Imperfect in an Imperfect World

WILLIAM G. BARTHOLOME

Over the last several years I have had the opportunity of doing a fair amount of public speaking. For reasons that are not all apparent to me, I have developed a habit of beginning most of those addresses with what is best called an apologia—a plea for understanding or sympathy or mercy.

I accepted this invitation at a point in my personal development that might best be characterized as a prolonged phase of *angry cynicism.* I think I have always been (and may well always be) angry. My anger is rarely focused at particular individuals. It is, I think, much like the anger of the doctor in Camus' *The Plague*—anger at God, at the human condition, at being called upon to live in an imperfect world. I find it to be relatively easy to accept imperfections in individual others, because I know myself to be imperfect. Yet, that level of imperfection still allows us to do right by each other. In our individual relationships with each other we can be moral men and women. The anger comes whenever I move beyond that level. My anger intensifies as I broaden my focus— from individuals to families, to organizations, to communities, to institutions, to cities, to states, etc.

My cynicism is of a much more recent onset. I have used my anger, frustration, and resentment much like an automobile uses gasoline, namely, as the fuel that allowed me to get where I am today. I have crammed my head full of what is called our accumulated knowledge through a prolonged educational and training process. I then took that education and training, accepted a position on a medical school faculty, and entered the fight. My fight might best be labeled a fight for the liberation of children, particularly handicapped or "deviant" children. The primary method I have employed is that of advocacy. In attempting to play that role for my own children, for my patients, for patients in our teaching hospitals, for children in residential settings, and for children as a class, I have repeatedly had to deal with children's professionals, schools, school systems, agencies, programs, and a host of other social agents, systems, and institutions. One result of those multiple encounters has been that I have become extremely cynical—I am (to quote Webster) contemptuously distrustful of social institutions and those who act as their agents.

My apologia, therefore, is that my remarks will be a reflection of my angry cynicism. I am asking that you attempt to understand. My apologia is also directly relevant to the topic I was given "Good Intentions become Imperfect in an Imperfect World." Dr. van Eys assures me that he chose the topic before he chose the speaker, but I wonder.

The word intention is interesting in that it has several radically different meanings or definitions. Since our conference is about "reintegration" of the child who has or has had cancer, I assume that in this context intentions are what we intend to do or to bring about, namely reintegration. The "good" intention is thus bringing about or causing it to happen that the child with cancer is reintegrated.

I will return to a very different definition of the word intention later. According to this alternative definition, intentions have less to do with achieving a state of affairs—reintegration—and more to do with a determination or resolve to act *in a certain way*, for example, one intends to act or behave courteously.

If reintegration is thus a state of affairs or a process by which some state of affairs is achieved, the claim that I am attempting to defend is that given that you and I and children with cancer live in an imperfect world, such a state of affairs will never be achieved, or that the process will be in some fundamental way imperfect, defective, or flawed.

Your first response might well be "so what?" As a matter of fact, everyone with whom I have shared the title of this paper (including myself) felt that such a claim was so trite or obvious that it bordered on a nonsense claim. It sounds a little bit like saying "If you try to carry water in a bucket with holes in the bottom, you'll lose some water." That may sound so obvious that it's silly, but if at this conference we are to look at how to achieve something, it may be essential to realize that all tools or methods at our disposal are flawed, imperfect. But that is not my claim.

Others have responded to my title by saying, "Is that the same as saying 'the road to hell is paved with good intentions?' " I can remember that my father was very enamored of that particular saying. I don't believe that's what I'm saying either. The road-to-hell claim is that if we want reintegration of the child with cancer, we need to do more than have good intentions, we need to act, to do something.

What I am trying to claim is that we should *not* make the mistake of believing that we can achieve a goal or state of affairs called reintegration of the child with cancer, even in an incomplete or less than perfect sense.

Your response might well be: "Well, if it can't be achieved, if our good intentions are fated to become imperfect, what are we doing here?" I hope that question will be addressed over the course of the conference. And, I think it's a very good question.

Let me continue. This is the Fifth Annual Mental Health Conference in this series. The focus of this series has become progressively wider. It began with a focus on the individual child with cancer and the claim that responding to such a child demanded of us a concern that was broader than the killing of malignant cells, that we must deal with a whole child. Since most children live in families, that concern quite naturally expands to include the child's siblings and parents. To provide even a very minimal level of care to the child, it was obvious that efforts had to be made to provide some level of support for the family. Following conferences in this series also focused on the creation of a special environment for the child under our care, on organizational concepts for the community of providers. This was expressed as "total patient care in a therapeutic community." One of the concepts that was used was that of the normally sick child—a pregnant and powerful metaphor (1).

Since the "good intentions" involved were focused on the child, the child's immediate family, and hospital and clinic staff and environment, the task, although extremely challenging and problematic, was in some sense double. Given the right kind of leadership and a highly dedicated and determined staff, the goal of providing care to normally sick children in a therapeutic community could be achieved. The fact that even this "good intention" requires an almost superhuman expenditure of time and effort is worth noting. Similarly, the child's home caretakers could be helped to see and respond to the child as normally sick and to render the home environment a more therapeutic one.

However, our focus here is radically different. That is what I think needs to be understood. I would argue that to get those outside the child's home and those outside the hospital-clinic environments to see and respond to the child as normally sick or to have the child's total environment be subsumed under the concept of a therapeutic community is not possible. We will need to discover different concepts. We will need to devise other strategies.

Why do I make this claim? Why is this project in some sense fated to fail?

First, we all need to realize the extent to which we are bound by our time and place. The idea of reintegration or what is more commonly called rehabilitation is a concept that has only recently emerged. In fact, the idea of working with the disabled or handicapped to help them "reach vocational and economic goals and social potential commensurate with their residual abilities" (2) was a revolutionary idea when it emerged in the mid-19th century. And after a very brief flurry of activity, the idea was virtually abandoned until after the Second World War. Although it may seem familiar to all of us who are professionals, it is a very new concept; we are all beginners, novices in terms of rehabilitation.

Second, it is essential for us as professionals to remind ourselves constantly of the differences between doing or achieving good and doing our duty, fulfilling our strict obligations to our patients/clients/students. (I should note that I will refer to the child with cancer as a patient. That is another reflection of my perspective. They are also for many of you "clients" or "students" or simply children.) In recent years there has developed in the helping professions, particularly within medicine, a debate between those who argue that the end or purpose of medicine is to cure, to heal, to restore patients to health, and a smaller group who argue that the end of medicine is to care, to fulfill our basic duties and obligations to patients, and to do no harm. For the latter group cure is seen as good and desirable, but not part of what we *owe* the patient. Patients may have rights in health care or possibly even to a minimum level of health care, but a right to health or to be made healthy is a very different concept. Unfortunately, one group has been labeled "disease oriented" and the other "person oriented." As a student of ethics, I would argue that those who hold that cure is primary are arguing that the professional is to judge himself and be judged using the yardstick of consequences, benefits. Doing good, conferring benefits is primary. Those who argue that care is primary are arguing that the professional is to judge himself and be judged using the yardstick of duty or obligation, duties like competence and obligations like truth telling. Doing right, for them, is prior to and more basic than doing good. I find myself firmly in the camp of this latter group. I would argue that the primary focus of the professional must be on doing right by the patient. If cure can be attained, if our patients can benefit from what we do, then that is clearly good; but we should not measure ourselves or be measured by how much good we can produce. My favorite example of why that is so is the case of the dying patient, but the same argument seems to apply to the chronically ill, the handicapped.

It is essential that we see the concept of reintegration as good, or a desirable goal for the children for whom we care. However, it is equally essential to argue that our efforts in this regard are not our basic duty or obligation to them. In *The Normally Sick Child*, Jan van Eys (1) made the claim, "By taking responsibility for the cure, we must also accept responsibility for the consequences." I would argue that this claim is problematic in two senses. First, I don't believe we have a responsibility to cure, but rather to provide the best care we can. Second, if treatment of the child with cancer is associated with a significant number of serious side effects or consequences, the responsibility of responding to these created problems, for example, an amputated leg, is a different kind of responsibility. If it is our belief that the best we can do for the patient is to amputate her leg, we owe that patient our good faith effort at helping her adjust to her new situation; but we do not owe her in the same sense that we would had one of us amputated her leg through negligence in, say, causing an automobile accident in which she lost a leg.

My third reason for the claim that the good intention of reintegration will become imperfect is highly pragmatic, of which I have three concerns. One deals with the labeling process, the second with Public Law 94-142 as an object lesson, and the third about the use of the goal of reintegration as a psychological avoidance mechanism. In ethics there is a long-standing argument that right implies can. It cannot be our duty or obligation to do what we cannot achieve. I would argue that reintegration of the child with cancer is an impossible ideal; however, that does not mean bad or wrong.

My first claim is that in some sense we have created and are the institutions that define and shape the social role "child with cancer." In other words, by our actions we segregate, we define, we label; we create a need for reintegration. That is not as bizarre as it might sound initially.

The child with cancer prior to about 1940 played the role of a dying child. Cure, even prolonged survival, was exceedingly rare. There were no children who wore the label child-with-cancer for longer than several months.

That situation has changed dramatically. What was once an almost universally fatal disease is now almost always a chronic disease. By our efforts we have created a new social role; there are now relatively large numbers of children who wear a new label. And although for some their label is relatively invisible from a social perspective, for most there are the combined scars of disease and treatment. Many, if not most, are handicapped in one way or another.

In a very real sense, we have created a population of children who from a social perspective are deviant (3); they are seen by others as different, not normal. And there is at least some evidence to support the claim that the label "cancer patient" is what sociologists have called a stigmatizing label (4). That is to say that the imputation of difference or deviance is not based on any behavioral or biological fact about the child, but largely based on fear, awe, prejudice, or ignorance. It has been argued that the treatment process itself and the language we use to describe it creates a distancing, a negative response in the community of persons around the child. Not only are cancer patients scary because they have cancer, but because they are treated in awesome research centers with highly dangerous and powerful drugs and radiation. They are removed for extended periods of time from the everyday world and taken up, almost like someone would be taken up by an alien space craft, to the incomprehensible world of the cancer center. If children with cancer could be taken care of by their local doctors with medicine you can get in the drug-store on the corner and hospitalized at the same place kids go to get hernias repaired or broken arms fixed, the extent of their perceived deviance would be diminished significantly.

As we concern ourselves with reintegration, we need to be aware of the extent to which we are, at least, one potent source of the problem.

My second pragmatic consideration, I would argue, is that reintegration is an impossible ideal simply because we cannot force the world to be a therapeutic community. Our patients not only face the world as children—a significantly stigmatizing label—but as handicapped children. The lesson that forcing social institutions to provide the handicapped with equality of opportunity may well be impossible is a lesson many of us are now learning. The best example and one that is very germane to our work is Public Law 94-142, otherwise known as the Education for All Handicapped Children Act of 1975 (5). Though of good intention, the law is deceptively simple in its goals. Through a free, public education, the handicapped child was to be helped to achieve "the basic minimum skills needed to exercise his/her constitutional rights" and a maximal degree of self-sufficiency or self-care. The basic principles are essentially three: a zero reject principle—no child is to be designated as uneducable; an appropriate educational experience (to preclude functionally excluding the child by inappropriate placement); and education in the least restrictive setting (also frequently called mainstreaming). The intent was to issue the mandate using the club of threats to cut off federal funding (about 10% of all monies spent in Texas on education) and to share the economic burden created by the legislation by gradually increasing the federal allocation from 5% of average pupil expense in 1978 to 40% by 1982. The cost was estimated to be approximately $400 million in 1978 and increasing to between $3 and $3.5 billion by 1982. The target population was an estimated 8 million (some 4–5 million of whom had already been identified) handicapped children between the ages of 3 and 21 years.

I would like to take a brief look at what happened to this good intention, say, in the state of Texas. About one in nine children in the U.S. live in Texas. In rough figures that's about five million children. If one assumes that between 10% and 12% of all children are handicapped, the target population in Texas is roughly 600,000. (Of that number at least half have a major disability and some 350,000 are identified and enrolled in special education programs.)

Texas spends a substantial sum of money each year on education, approximately half of the state budget. And roughly 50% of public school money comes from the state. However, expenditures for public education in Texas are significantly different from those in other states. Texans are generous almost without parallel in their support of graduate and professional students. Texas spends more per student in professional schools than any state in the country except California (though Proposition 13 will no doubt change that). College students are also generously supported — Texas ranks in the top ten. But in terms of expenditures for elementary and secondary school students, Texas ranks 39 out of 50 (6). We spend less than $1,000 per year per student (and in many areas of the state less than $500 per year per student) to educate elementary and secondary school students. As a result, most school districts in the state relied heavily on contractual arrangements with private foundations, agencies, and schools for providing service to handicapped children, and excluded or at least didn't serve many severely handicapped children at all. That was particularly the case for school districts in large cities such as Houston.

These contractual arrangements also had effects beyond the economic issues. Handicapped children were segregated from the public school system. Since special education programs were administered at a level above the individual school principal and usually conducted in separate schools, buildings, or at contracting facilities, the school system was insulated from the handicapped student. Few teachers had training or experience in working with the handicapped. Since most programs and contracting facilities provided categorial services, even special education teachers had limited training or experience with the broad range of handicapping conditions. A given special education teacher might know a great deal about, for example, educational needs and methods for a child with cerebral palsy, but know little or nothing about education of the blind or deaf child. One can readily appreciate the panic and resentment of the Houston Independent School District elementary school teacher—paid less than an unskilled laborer, faced with the day-in and day-out task of attempting to teach 30–35 socially disadvantaged children—who is now told that in addition she must respond to the needs of a child with a severe reading disorder *and* a child with myelodysplasia who is chairbound *and* a child with a significant hearing problem *and* a child with significant emotional problems.

The law also seems to have assumed a level of expertise in determining "appropriate education" that most consider fanciful. Hard, reliable information about child development is by and large less than 25 years old; reliable information about the development and needs of the handicapped child is not only new, but often sketchy and unreliable. Congress seems to have had little appreciation of how ambiguous and uncertain the enterprise of special education actually is (7).

The law mandates that every child receive an extensive evaluation and it assumes that there is some objective, reliable yardstick by which this can be done in a nonbiased, culture-free manner. These tools are in their infancy and the use of even the most widely accepted measurement tools is highly controversial.

The law also mandates that the school provide a wide array of services within the school that have rarely been part of special education programs in the public school, speech pathology and audiology, psychological services, physical and occupational therapy, and medical and counseling services. Most teachers were educated to expect that these were, in most cases, extracurricular services. Few school districts have huge cadres of such professionals on their staffs. There are also few training programs in such professions that include comprehensive training in the care of the handicapped child (8).

The lawmakers also failed to deal adequately with several major concentrations of power and authority in education. The Texas Education Agency, which has an established reputation for only acting if forced into a corner, submitted a plan for implementation of Public Law 94-142 to the Bureau of Education of the Handicapped, which they knew made a mockery of the law. Their plan required some 80 revisions to even approximate an adequate plan and their obstructionism resulted in a delay in $72 million of federal support for three quarters of 1979.

Then there are school boards and principals. School boards in Texas have historically paid little more than lip service to the educational needs of the handicapped. The new law calls for an impartial hearing process to adjudicate irreconcilable conflicts between parents and the school system. However, local school boards have been very reluctant to allow hearing officers the authority to ask for changes in a district program to meet the needs of a handicapped child. Principals have almost unlimited authority in terms of what happens at individual schools. They have historically seen special education as someone else's job, but the law threatens the time honored distinction between regular and special education. It asks that children with problems receive education on what the principal feels is her turf. Yet, many principals have been openly hostile to these changes. The cry "Why should I ask that my staff change what they are doing for 90–95% of students in order that a small number of handicapped can get what they want?" indicates either an unwillingness or inability to feel the force of the demand for an end to discrimination on the basis of handicap.

Although the long-term outcome of this "good intention" remains to be seen and a total condemnation of the program is premature, it is safe to say that the overall impact to date has been largely negative. Many parents and educators feel that a whole generation of handicapped children will be the unwitting subjects of this very risky social experiment. Several commentators have referred to Public Law 94-142 as the full employment act for attorneys. And most commentators believe that the act has severely strained the relationship between parents and the educational system (9).

Parents, many of whom had children in private, categorical programs under contract with the school system, are demanding that the school do at least as much for their child as was being done previously—a not unreasonable demand. School districts are caught in an economic crunch and the promised federal subsidy has not been forthcoming. It is widely assumed that given the present state of the economy, the federal share of costs will not increase beyond the present budgeted level of 10% at least for the next two or three years. The funding of public education at a local level via property taxes has come under increasing attack. It is highly unlikely that districts will be able to get public support for the sharp increase in expenditures required to do the task. In the meantime, the private organizations and agencies that had provided services are being stripped of personnel and financial support to the extent that even their short-term survival is in question.

The overall result has been the development of a massive amount of frustration, anger, and cynicism. And as parents turn to the legal system and the courts to force compliance for their individual child, and demand formal hearings as a matter of course, the whole enterprise begins to topple. Huge sums of money and significant amounts of staff time and effort are wasted trying to defend the system from parents who are seen and being forced to behave as adversaries. Parents who are less well informed and cannot afford the emotional and financial costs involved in forcing compliance find that their children often receive "in name only" services. To defend the system from the threat of a loss of federal funds, districts are forced to spend a significant amount of time and energy on demonstrating at least "paper compliance" with the mandate. It is exceedingly difficult for me to see that my patients and their families have benefitted from the new law. I am also pessimistic about at least the short-term effects of the law on the education of the handicapped.

Although our patients are rarely severely handicapped, they join the ranks of the 300,000–400,000 involved in this chaos. What happens to our goal of reintegration? Will we be able to force the system to meet their special needs? The cynic in me wants to say "only if we provide them legal services." And even that is no guarantee. It is—to quote another of my father's favorites—hard to get blood from a turnip.

My third pragmatic concern is that the good intention of having our patients be reintegrated may well have a subtle evil effect on our treatment of children with cancer. If we, as Doctor van Eys suggests (1), are willing to accept responsibility for the consequences of our efforts to cure and to obligate ourselves to reintegrate our handicapped-by-treatment patients into society, this psychological game can be used to help us avoid confrontation with the underbelly, the shadow side, the ambiguous and often tragic aspects of what we do with our treatments. If there is such a thing as an obligation to do research, I would argue that the highest priority for research on a significant number of malignant diseases of children must be given to research aimed at decreasing the costs of treatment to the child. A willingness to accept responsibility for having chopped off John's leg and a willingness to try to reintegrate this now handicapped person into society are both cheap. One of my biggest problems with those who would expand the concept of responsibility in medicine is that it's frequently hard for me to see what the patients gain from our willingness to accept the responsibility for what we have done to them.

If we see reintegration as a readily attainable goal—a goal no different in principle from our previous goal of holistic care of the normally sick child in a therapeutic community—we run the risk of blinding ourselves to the highly ambiguous and tragic work we do. We run the risk of deceiving ourselves and the children we feel called to serve.

Let me summarize. I have argued that we must see our good intentions of reintegration of the child with cancer as impossible, imperfect. I argued that the previous concept of the normally sick child and the therapeutic community will not stretch across the huge chasm between home/hospital and the world outside; that we need to be aware that the reintegration-rehabilitation movement is in its infancy; that reintegration should not be defined as our duty to patients in the strict sense, that is to say, that our primary duty is to render care in a manner respectful of our normally sick patients and of ourselves as a community of providers. I then listed what I feel are three basically pragmatic concerns: First, that by virtue of a kind of catch-22 we have generated the problem we seek to address—we have created the deviant social role, child-with-cancer, we take them up into our institutions and label them. Second, social justice, equality of opportunity, is an exceedingly difficult (if not impossible) ideal. In Public Law 94-142 we have an excellent object lesson in how good intentions become imperfect. And third, that a focus on reintegration may well divert our efforts to reduce the handicaps induced by our efforts to cure.

Some of you will no doubt be puzzled. It sounds as if I am saying that those who organized this conference and brought all of us together have made a mistake; you may be hearing me say that a concern, a good intention about our patients and students, namely, reintegration, is wrong or misguided.

What I am trying to say is that we need to be wary, doubtful, even cynical. We need to realize that although it would be a very good thing, reintegration in any complete sense will not be achieved. If we accept this demand on us, we need to be aware that it is an impossible demand. We will need to develop a new and different strategy and new and different concepts.

I would like to close with what I think may be concepts or ideas worth exploring. If we admit that perfect justice cannot be achieved, we are faced with developing a concept of imperfect justice. If the idea of reintegration is to serve as a beacon that will guide our efforts, we need to develop a plan, to chart a course through the imperfect world in which we live.

I would suggest that we might find it helpful to accept the fact that the child with cancer facing the world beyond hospital/clinic and home will be seen and responded to as a social deviant, that he will wear a stigmatizing label. As I wrote these remarks I was reminded of an experience I had working in the clinic at Johns Hopkins Hospital in Baltimore. I was interviewing a six-year-old black child who had been brought to see me about a problem he was having at school. As he and I attempted to talk with one another, he was constantly interrupted by his mother's instructions to answer my questions "yes, sir" and "no, sir." After several minutes of this frustrating conversation I turned to his mother and explained to her that I would rather her son simply respond to my questions and that I saw no need of his accompanying each response with "sir." After several visits during which the mother continued to closely monitor and constantly correct her son's responses to me, I elected to set up a visit with mom alone.

In the course of our visit, this mother defended her behavior by pointing out to me that even though I felt her son's self-effacing "sirring" was inappropriate, she felt it was essential. Her claim was: "a good black mother gotta teach her babies how to behave 'round whitey.'" She shared my dream that her child might someday be integrated into society, but she knew all to well that in the here and now black children needed to be prepared to deal with racism as their daily fare, as something to be expected in dealings with "whitey."

I think that a major focus of our concern should be on teaching our patients and students to deal with the prejudice, ignorance, and fear in others that they will encounter. We need to train them in how to "pass" for normal when that is the best strategy; how to "cover" their deviance so as to keep it from intruding on social intercourse; and how to reduce the tension in the encounter with "normals." We need to train them in how to make people immediately and fully aware of the deviance when "pass" or "cover" won't work.

I think we must also provide training for parents and siblings in how to work the system, how to get the system to respond, however reluctantly, to the special needs of their child. We need to not only help the parents cope with their own problems in having a handicapped, a deviant child, but to get them as rapidly as possible to a place where they can become radical advocates for their child. It is clear to most child advocates that the teeth, the driving force behind Public Law 94-142 was the crucial power and authority delegated to parents. A handicapped child, by and large, will get little or nothing more than her parents demand of the system. That few parents are informed enough or strong enough to play this role effectively is a remediable problem.

I think we also need to consider the idea of the case manager or ombudsman or outside advocate. The crucial aspect of this limited program of reintegration is the perceived reality of the child (10). If the child feels that she can effectively deal with deviance in social intercourse, we are at least on course. The problem is that to know what's going on inside the child, we need to provide each child with someone who will maintain an intimate, open, and honest relationship over a prolonged period of time. Obviously, the primary individuals who will play this role are the parents. However, I wonder if there needs to be an additional person from the provider community who will play the role.

And finally, you may remember that I said that the word intention has more than one meaning. I have argued that good intentions become imperfect in an imperfect world; that is the case if intentions are defined as something we intend to do, to bring about, a state of affairs—like equality of opportunity or reintegration. The other meaning of the word intention is that an intention is a determination, a resolve to act in a particular way, like I intend to act or behave courteously. If our good intention is a resolve, a determination, a dedication, a willingness to fight, to struggle, regardless of the ultimate success or failure of our efforts, a good intention need not become imperfect. But remember that's the kind that "paves the road to hell."

I think that reintegration is not a state of affairs that can be achieved; it is an impossible ideal that calls us to do battle, to fight for and with our patients, though we fight in a struggle that we all know will never end.

REFERENCES

1. van Eys, J., ed. The Normally Sick Child. Baltimore: University Park Press, 1979.
2. Rosen, M., Clark, G., Kivitz, M. Habilitation of the Handicapped. Baltimore: University Park Press, 1977.
3. Freidson, E. Disability as social deviance. In: Freidson, E., ed. Medical Men and Their Work. New York: Aldine, 1972.
4. Goffman, E. Stigma: Notes on the Management of Spoiled Identity. New Jersey: Spectrum Books, 1963.
5. Education for All Handicapped Children Act of 1975. Public Law 94-142, 29 Nov. 1975, 89 STAT. 773-96: Federal Register 42(163): 42474-518, 23 Aug. 1977.
6. Watson, J. Still the Darker Side of Childhood. Austin, Tex: Texas Department of Community Affairs, 1978.
7. Palfrey, J., et al. New Directions in the evolution and education of handicapped children. N. Engl. J. Med., 289:819–824, 19.
8. Jacobs, F., Walker, D. Pediatrics and the Education for All Handicapped Children Act of 1975. Pediatrics, 61:135–137, 1978.
9. Educating all handicapped children: A review of progress and problems. Amicus, 4:67–95, 1979.
10. Travis, G. Chronic Illness in Children. Stanford, Calif: Stanford University Press, 1976, pp. 43–74.

Section II
THE REALITY

Introduction

ROSE HICKS

Lest we allow ourselves to think that Public Law 94-142 sprung forth from the Federal Government without warning, let me explore the etiology of this and other similar legislation. Let's move back in time to World War I; how many soldiers, injured in battle, lived? How many babies survived through infantile diseases? Not many. Just remember where we were at that time in medicine and technology. Where in the history of medicine were we during the World War II period? We were coming along. More of the injured survived, but many were handicapped as a result of their injury. They could no longer hold the job that they once had. Society denied them a reentry into the mainstream of life. Some of the denial was nonverbal; the looks, the stares, the pity, the rank of second class citizen. Additionally, schools, churches, and theaters, once accessible to these people, were no longer accessible because of the special mobility equipment they required. Yet they were needed in society. The Korean War came and went and the problems magnified. As problems arose and were solved with the handicapped veterans, society became aware of handicapped children and their needs. There are ever more such children as modern medicine learns to cure at a price. Yet so much could be accomplished if we just accepted the presence of potential in these children. Attorney Dayle Bebee will address the laws affecting the handicapped in the schools, dealing with their history, definition, and application. Doctor Betty Pfefferbaum will address the reintegration of the handicapped.

CHAPTER 3

The Right to Education for Handicapped Children

DAYLE BEBEE

Incredible as it may seem, the right to an education for a handicapped child is a concept that has only recently become a reality. In the 1970s when Congress began studying the idea of providing an education to the handicapped children in our nation, the surprising facts appeared in a congressional report:

> Without adequate education, individuals with handicaps are doomed to a continued life as 2nd-class citizens. Today our country is only educating 40% of those individuals with handicaps. Sixty percent of these individuals are receiving a substandard education. (1)

In this paper I will review the very recent developments that are making education a reality for handicapped children: the pioneering court decisions that have now borne fruit in new federal legislative enactments mandating an education for the handicapped child.

In 1954 the United States Supreme Court made the following declarations in the case *Brown* v. *Board of Education.* (2):

> Today education is perhaps the most important function of state and local governments. Compulsory school attendance laws and the great expenditures for education both demonstrate our recognition of the importance of education to our democratic society. It is required in the performance of our most basic public responsibilities, even service in the armed

forces. It is the very foundation of good citizenship. Today it is a principle instrument in awakening the child to cultural values, in preparing him for later professional training, and in helping him to adjust normally to his environment. In these days, it is doubtful that any child may reasonably be expected to succeed in life if he is denied the opportunity of an education. Such an opportunity, where the state has undertaken to provide it, is a right which must be made available to all on equal terms.

That is a beautiful statement about education in our country, but the Supreme Court was talking specifically about Negro children in that case, and handicapped children were not entitled to the benefit of those guarantees until almost 20 years later.

The landmark case of *Pennsylvania Association of Retarded Citizens* v. *Commonwealth of Pennsylvania* (3) was decided in 1972, only eight years ago. In that case the principle of equal educational opportunity was applied to all mentally retarded children in Pennsylvania. The three-judge panel held:

Without exception expert opinion indicates that: All mentally retarded persons are capable of benefiting from a program of education and training, that the greatest number of retarded persons, given such education and training, are capable of achieving some degree of self care; that the earlier such education and training begins, the more thoroughly and the more efficiently a mentally retarded person will benefit from it and whether begun early or not, that a mentally retarded person can benefit at any point in his life and development from a program of education. (3)

These mentally retarded children had been excluded from an education by the state on the grounds that they could not be expected to benefit from education. The public school officials were ordered to provide every mentally retarded child access to a free public program of education and training, and to provide notice, opportunity for a hearing, and periodic reevaluation regarding any change in educational status. Thus, for the first time, it was made clear that not only were the mentally retarded children entitled to a free public education, but that certain procedural safeguards must be provided to insure the proper implementation of that right to an education—a milestone in the lives of mentally retarded children.

Shortly following the *Pennsylvania Association for Retarded Citizens* case, a federal court extended these rights to all handicapped children in *Mills* v. *Board of Education of the District of Columbia* (4). This was a class-action suit brought on behalf of Washington, D.C. school-age children who, though eligible for education, had been denied placement in the District's publicly supported educational programs because of alleged mental, behavioral, physical, or emotional handicaps or deficiencies. The plaintiff children had been suspended or expelled from school programs without being offered a hearing and without being provided alternative educational placements.

In its extremely detailed opinion, the court found that the District of Columbia Public School System had an affirmative duty, under D.C. statutes, to provide plaintiffs and their class with publicly supported, specialized instruction suited to each child's needs. The court also found that the plaintiffs' right to a suitable education was guaranteed by the due process clause of the fifth amendment.

The public school system's practice of reassigning, suspending, or expelling handicapped children from regular school programs or specialized instruction without any prior hearing and no subsequent periodic review violated the due process clause. "Due process of law requires that each child be afforded a hearing prior to exclusion, termination [or] classification into a special program." (4)

The court rejected outright the defendants' claim that insufficient funds excused their failure to "include and retain these children in the public school system, or otherwise provide them with publicly supported education and ... to afford them due process hearings and periodic service." (4) The court responded that if sufficient funds are truly not available,

> then the available funds must be expended equitably in such a manner that no child [whether handicapped or non-handicapped] is entirely excluded from a publicly supported education consistent with his needs and ability to benefit therefrom. ... The inadequacies of the District of Columbia Public School System whether occasioned by insufficient funding or administrative inefficiency, certainly cannot be permitted to bear more heavily on the 'exceptional' or handicapped child than on the normal child. (4)

The court's order adopted the proposition that every child, no matter how severe the handicap, is educable and must receive suitable publicly supported instruction:

> The District of Columbia shall provide to each child of school-age a free and suitable publicly supported education regardless of the degree of the child's mental, physical or emotional disability or impairment. (4)

Consequently, a handicapped child may not be excluded from a regular public school assignment without receiving at public expense an adequate and immediate alternative educational placement or tuition grants, consistent with the child's needs.

The court ordered the public school system to provide for a due process adversary hearing for handicapped children's parents or guardians to contest the school's proposed action affecting their children's educational placement. Parents and guardians must be offered an opportunity for a due process hearing: before initial placement, denial of placement, or change of placement of a handicapped child in a special education program; and before the school proposes to take disciplinary measures that will exclude, suspend, postpone, transfer, or otherwise deny access to the regular school program to a handicapped child.

The opinion in the *Mills* case goes into great detail about the notice that must go out to parents, about the hearing procedures that must be followed, and about the use of disciplinary procedures.

This brings us, then, to the beginning of a recognition by Congress of the right to a free, public education for handicapped children. In 1974 Congress responded by enacting Public Law 93-380 (5), amended in 1975 by Public Law 94-142, the Education for All Handicapped Children Act (6). Both laws specifically recognize that it is the public policy of the United States of America that every citizen is entitled to an education to meet his or her full potential without financial barriers.

Immediately prior to these enactments, Congress passed into law the Vocational Rehabilitation Act of 1973 (7), which prohibits recipients of federal funds (including public education systems) from discriminating against otherwise qualified handicapped persons. It is clear that Section 504 forbids discrimination in public education on the grounds of a person's handicap to the same extent that the Civil Rights Act of 1964 forbids discrimination on the basis of race or national origin.

Thus, the combined effect of Section 504 of the Rehabilitation Act and Public Law 94-142 is that federal law recognizes the right of handicapped children to equal access to public school education programs. However, this is only now in 1980 becoming a reality.

REFERENCES

1. 74 U. S. Code Congress and Ad. News 6407.
2. *Brown* v. *Board of Education*, 347 U. S. 483, 74 Supreme Court 686, 98 L. Ed. 873 (1954).
3. *Pennsylvania Association for Retarded Citizens* v. *Commonwealth of Pennsylvania*, 334 F. Supp. 1257 (E. D. Pa. 1971) and 343 F. Supp. 279 (E. D. Pa. 1972).

4. *Mills* v. *Board of Education of District of Columbia,* 348 F. Supp. 866 (D. D. C. 1972).
5. Education of the Handicapped Act, 20 U. S. C. 821, 88 Stat. 484 (1974).
6. Education for All Handicapped Children Act, 20 U. S. C. 1401 (1975).
7. Vocational Rehabilitation Act, 29 U. S. C. 794 (1973).

CHAPTER 4

Reintegration of the Handicapped

BETTY PFEFFERBAUM

"What fine ducklings," the old Grandmother said. "But why waste your time sitting on that large egg any longer. I'm sure it's a turkey's egg and a little turkey is a great bother to a duck. . . ."

The next day the large egg cracked and out came the strangest looking duck she had ever seen. Instead of being yellow and fluffy like the other ducklings, it was an ugly greenish gray color and it had a long neck and long, awkward legs.

"He's the ugliest child I ever had," thought Mother Duck. But she treated him kindly and tried not to let him feel that he was different from the others. . . .

But Mother Duck could not be beside the Ugly Duckling all the time, and whenever she was away from him for a moment, someone teased him or pecked at him. The Ugly Duckling was given no peace. Even his own brothers and sisters made fun of him, and the girl who came out to feed them kicked him away.

Day after day things grew worse. The Ugly Duckling was treated so badly that he decided to run away. He ran toward the fence, spreading his wings, and by using all his strength he managed to fly over it. The little birds in the bushes where he landed flew away in fright. "That is because I am so ugly that I terrified them," he thought sadly (1).

This well known children's story depicts the fate of the ugly duckling who, because he was different, was ostracized by society. The subject of this conference deals with children who, like the ugly duckling, may be ostracized because of their differences. These children are handicapped. For the sake of discussion, we may include under handicapped any physical illness that is of a chronic nature or that produces continuous strife and extraordinary demands for coping. For example, this may include an acute illness that results in hearing loss, blindness, amputation, or brain damage. A handicapped child may suffer from a primary psychological or psychiatric problem as, for example, those children with developmental disabilities. Or the handicapped child may suffer psychosocial or educational sequelae secondary to a primary disorder or its treatment.

An examination of the literature reveals the scope of the problem. The rate of chronic illness in the general pediatric population is reported at between 5% and 20%. The incidence of behavioral, psychological, and educational sequelae are generally reported as higher in the chronic-illness population than in the general population. The frequency of behavioral symptomatology is directly related to the duration of the illness and to the severity of the handicap assessed in terms of interference with activities of daily living (2). The nature of the relationship between impairment and psychosocial adjustment remains somewhat vague and perhaps varies with different disorders. Nonetheless, the psychological, social, and educational status of the handicapped child warrants attention.

Treatment often requires removing the child from his usual environment. Reintegration concerns itself with the movement of the child from a treatment setting into the mainstream of the family and social life both during and after treatment. The concept of reintegration reflects the concern that the status and needs of the handicapped set them apart from their age mates so that they fail to receive the usual array of social and educational services.

Need for reintegration stems from segregation, which may exist for several reasons. Illness and treatment may impel a child to avoid social interaction. The incidence of school phobia in children with chronic illness is high. It has been reported as high as 10% in some pediatric cancer populations (3). This compares with an incidence of 1.7% per year in the general school-age population (4). In some instances the handicapped children are removed from the usual school and social situations and given special, separate attention. This may be promoted by parents, health care providers, educators, and the general citizenry.

There is a natural tendency historically to segregate any persons perceived as "different." As indicated earlier this is not always imposed from without. All too often one finds the child isolating herself because of depression, fear of rejection, or unfamiliarity. Also too often, however, this isolation is fostered by overprotective parents, apprehensive school personnel, and thoughtless, frightened peers.

Coincident with segregation is labeling. Labeling allows separation and separation encourages labeling. A label, like a diagnosis, may imply prognosis, goals, and treatment approaches. In many instances this promotes care. However, when a diagnosis is not accompanied with a treatment plan, there is realistic concern that it serves only the purpose of labeling. Labeling reinforces negative attitudes and may prescribe the nature of social interaction. Labeling then has the potential of being detrimental. This may happen in a number of ways: by reducing the child to a single dimension, by emphasizing weaknesses, by reinforcing dependencies, by denying the opportunity for risk taking, and by perpetuating segregation and prejudice.

A label that initially may be used to describe one quality of a person becomes synonymous with all aspects of that person. The handicapped child then is more easily dismissed as a "diabetic," a "hemophiliac," or a "funny looking kid," and treated less as an individual and more as an anomaly.

Most often the tendency is to label a weakness rather than a strength. Even when a child is described as "special" or "exceptional," the negative aspect of the euphemism is soon fully comprehended. Labels declare expectations. Challenges for behavior and achievement are determined, in part at least, by expectations for success. Children actually perform or are credited with performing at the level of expectation.

The child himself may easily grow into his label. He begins to regard himself as others regard him, his self-concept and body image being reflections of the reactions of those around him. The standards by which he measures himself are learned.

Another natural consequence of labeling is the tendency to reinforce dependency. If the child is not given opportunities to try out her coping abilities, she has no test for her competence or endurance. Personality development requires the opportunity to face new challenges that encourage the development of coping or defense mechanisms. Encouraging the child to remain in or return to the mainstream places her in repeated situations that call for the development of adaptive skills. Frustration forces the child to find solutions. The demands for coping enhance the child's coping ability. Protecting the handicapped child from the cruelties of the environment does not allow her the opportunity to prepare for the numerous situations she is bound to face. Resiliency must be learned. The crises promoting development are the milestones of that development.

In the same vein, every individual deserves the opportunity to take risks. One is not required always to succeed. In fact, personality development requires the experience of failure. Everyone needs to be granted the chance to fail and to experience pain. No one is served by being shielded from the perplexities or pain of his condition. Failure must be tolerated and the child's need to suffer his own pain and build his own resources must be respected. If allowed to meet these challenges in a supportive, accepting environment, security and self-respect may become features of the self-concept.

Labeling perpetuates segregation. Prejudice, in part at least, stems from lack of exposure and familiarity and reinforces labeling and segregation.

Recognizing the dual concerns that some handicapped children never avail themselves of public services and that some are provided with special separate services, integration, at least in the educational sphere, has been mandated. The process is referred to as "mainstreaming" or "normalization." But just as labeling and segregation have shortcomings, so does normalization.

Integration in itself does not equal acceptance. Attitudes shape behavior. However, changes in behavior do not necessarily reflect changes in attitude. Do attitudes change just because a child with a handicap is placed in the same classroom with other children? Certainly physical integration alone does not insure acceptance. This has been learned from repeated attempts at racial integration and attempts at integrating the mentally ill and mentally retarded.

Chess et al. described the handicapped child in terms of "goodness of fit" to the environment. "Optimal development will occur to the extent that an organism's abilities, temperament and motivational patterns occur in a consonant interaction with the expectations and demands of the environment. Where there is dissonance between these environmental features and the organism's characteristics, resultant developmental and behavioral patterns may be suboptimal and/or pathologic." (5) The expectations and reactions within the family and the child's social and educational spheres help determine the child's adaptation.

Approaching the issue of reintegration from the various points on a time line allows an examination of problems apt to occur. First, at the time of diagnosis, the child and family may suffer shock and disbelief. Illness often demands removel for treatment purposes and naturally elicits protectiveness from parents. Care may be taken in early illness and treatment days to prevent psychosocial maladaptation later. Certainly, reintegration is made easier if the handicapped child is never far removed from her usual environment. If the child is capable of continued adaptation within the usual environment, she may never even require reintegration. One girl was observed from infancy, after the surgical removal of a retinoblastoma resulted in the loss of an eye. During the subsequent course of chemotherapy, a health care provider was heard to question the mother, "How long has your baby been ill?" The mother replied, "My daughter is not ill. She had cancer but that has been removed." By insisting early in the course of the illness that the child was to be considered normal, the mother paved the way for her daughter to establish a positive self-concept that would and did encourage the little girl to approach life without hesitancy about succeeding, but with a genuine knowledge of and respect for her physical limitations.

Some might argue that handicaps present since infancy pose less serious problems for the development of a positive self-concept and psychological adjustment. Consider another example, a disease such as cancer or diabetes that may present during childhood with acute and chronic components. The child may require removal from his usual milieu for an initial evaluation or during acute episodes. In this instance he is best approached with honesty and straightforwardness and encouraged to remain in or return to the mainstream. In this way the child learns resiliency early and comes to view the acute illness and treatment phases as intermittent obstacles to be overcome in a normal or more nearly normal developmental path. One 12-year-old with a five-year history of leukemia continued to insist that she be treated like her age mates even after treatment for her illness resulted in seizures and learning difficulties. Prior to the onset of these secondary problems she had lived as normally as possible despite extensive treatment and numerous hospitalizations. She was unwilling to relinquish the position of *acting* "normal" even if at times she did not *feel* "normal."

A final concern expressed with respect to normalization is that as a concept it may fail to take into account the importance of individual differences. It is as though anything "different" from the norm is negative. Being different is equated with being bad.

Current legislation mandating normalization focuses on individualization. Each handicapped child is expected to have an individual education program with special attention paid to her particular needs. This program may take into consideration the opinions of medical personnel as well as school personnel so that comprehensive management is provided. Just how successful the schools will be in implementing this legislation remains to be seen, for as previously indicated, some of the most important aspects of integration such as acceptance by others cannot be mandated.

MacMillan et al. discuss some of the problems associated with reintegration of the mildly retarded (6). The issues are not dissimilar in the handicapped population in general. First, the principle of reintegration must be distinguished from its implementation. To believe in an idea does not insure that the goal of the idea will be achieved. The school's and the society's sophistication, techniques, and materials necessary to implement the mandated reintegration need to be assessed. The success or failure of reintegration depends on the personalities, attitudes, and behaviors of those individuals directly involved in implementation. The willingness and preparation of school personnel cannot be assumed and the lack of willingness and preparation may be covertly expressed and may be more damaging than segregation itself. If the implementation fails, some may interpret the failure as evidence of a faulty principle and prejudices may become more deeply ingrained. There also is concern that one rigid model not be replaced by an equally rigid one. Even though individual planning is called for in reintegration, if the needs for such individualization are not realized, the end result may be as disastrous as segregation. Finally and most important, the child himself must be considered, for it is for his benefit that reintegration is mandated and it is his reaction and his growth that must be assessed in determining the value and effects of this approach.

In summary, the realistic problems of reintegration have been addressed. They include problems of resistance on the part of the child herself, on the part of concerned and sometimes overprotective family members, on the part of educators, and on the part of an already biased society at large. It is difficult to imagine a society in which labeling does not occur. Unfortunately, all ugly ducklings do not emerge from their crises as swans. Nonetheless, each deserves the right to struggle with her own crises and in that way to help predict the course of her own growth. Ultimately the children themselves will provide the means of critical assessment of this approach.

REFERENCES

1. Piper, W., ed. The ugly duckling. In: Stories That Never Grow Old. New York: Platt & Munk, 1969, pp. 9-16.
2. Pless, I. B., Roghmann, K. J. Chronic illness and its consequences: Observations based on three epidemiologic surveys. J. Pediatr., 79:351–359, 1971.
3. Lansky, S. B., Lowman, J. T., Vats, T., Gyulay, J. School phobia in children with malignant neoplasms. Am. J. Dis. Child., 129:42–46, 1975.
4. Kennedy, W. A. School phobia: Rapid treatment of fifty cases. J. Abnorm. Psychol., 70:285–289, 1965.
5. Chess, S., Fernandez, P., Korn, S. The handicapped child and his family: Consonance and dissonance. J. Am. Acad. Child Psychiatry, 19:56–67, 1980.
6. MacMillan, D. L., Jones, R. L., Myers, C. E. Mainstreaming the mildly retarded: Some questions, cautions and guidelines. Ment. Retard., 14: 3–10, 1976.

CHAPTER 5

The Reality of Reintegration of the Medically Exceptional Child — A Legal Viewpoint

DENNIS L. COBURN
BETTY PFEFFERBAUM

Following the plenary session on "The Reality," discussion groups focused on the legal liabilities and mandates surrounding the reintegration of the medically exceptional child. Initially, much concern was expressed about the liability of school personnel who perform medical procedures, such as catheterization, physical positioning, treatment of seizures, suctioning, and similar procedures. There was special concern about the possibilities of charges of negligence brought against them.

Discussion next turned to the area of the school's responsibility. Its most obvious responsibility is educating children; less obvious is its responsibility for facilitating children's participation in the educational process in the school. This second responsibility requires that the child's physician and the school cooperatively determine the role that each would play in assisting the student to be reintegrated.

If schools are to assist children in reintegration by providing educational services appropriate to meet their educational needs, then the various school programs of which a student may avail himself should be identified, as well as any eligibility criteria the student must meet. When speaking of students with medical disabilities, special education is the primary program. In determining eligibility for these programs, however, it was noted that medical definitions of "handicaps" and legal eligibility definitions of "handicaps" frequently do not coincide. And if a child is determined to be handicapped and eligible for special education on the basis of a temporary condition, is it in the child's best interest to be known as handicapped? If it is decided that such "labeling" should occur, then attention must be given to the removal of that label when the child's eligibility for special education no longer exists. Attention should also be given to protecting the child from any treatment as a handicapped person when he is no longer handicapped.

Two "threads" exist in any discussion of educating children who have medical problems. The first "thread" is providing an appropriate public education for the student whose medical problem constitutes an educational handicap and makes the student eligible for special education services. Public Law 94-142, the Education of All Handicapped Children Act, is specific for this population of students. It specifies the school's responsibilities for providing appropriate educational services (in the form of the Individualized Education Program) and for protecting the child's rights through procedural safeguards. A committee of professionals representing assessment (possibly medical and educational), instruction, and school administration are required to meet with the parents to draw up an educational program for a handicapped student, which takes into account the child's medical problems, so that the effect on the child's education is minimized.

This same or a comparable committee is required to meet at least every three months to review the child's progress and make any changes in the educational program that seems warranted. In addition, a triannual reevaluation is required to determine the child's continuing eligibility for special education services. The fact that the instruments used to measure those factors that would reflect educational handicaps are not totally accurate or reliable would indicate even more emphatically that determination of eligibility cannot be made by any one person. Such determinations should be made by a group of concerned professionals and the parents, exercising their best judgment in determining collaborative skills in assessing the various needs of the child and appropriate responses to those needs.

A second "thread" focuses on those students whose problems do not constitute an educational handicap, but who run the risk of developing educational handicaps as a secondary problem. The concern here is prevention of these secondary problems. There is no law that mandates schools to provide preventive services. Schools are, however, required to provide mainstream (non-special education) teachers with information and skilled training needed for working with children who have various problems constituting a handicap. It is hoped that such training will work to assist teachers in preventing children with medical problems from developing secondary educational handicaps.

Two particular populations of children were identified who present particular problems for the educator: The child who is removed from the school and hospitalized for medical reasons, and the child who is emotionally disturbed.

For the hospital child, the issue of continuing education both on hospital entry and discharge is necessary and difficult to achieve. School issues may be of low priority when the child is medically ill because the child is too sick to avail herself of educational services. If, however, the educational process is not realized, the child is likely to lose those skills she had and make reentry into a school classroom even more difficult. While the child is in the hospital, the emphasis is on keeping her from falling behind, that is, on maintaining her educational levels.

The emotionally disturbed child, removed from the regular classroom because of emotional problems, has needs similar to those children hospitalized for medical reasons. The problem of serving these children in school programs is exaggerated by the social deviance of the behaviors, which often is considered to be under control of the child. This frequently results in the child's being viewed as "bad" rather than "handicapped."

At this point a system exists for making educational services available in the hospital setting for these populations of students. The same system can be used to facilitate the child's return to the school program without disrupting the continuity of educational or medical services.

In some children, the trauma of being removed from school for medical or emotional reasons may be especially pronounced. Such an event may cause the child to be especially susceptible to developing secondary school problems. In such cases, there needs to be a set of services that can be utilized to diminish the child's susceptibility to the problem of transition. The system, i.e., the ARD Committee, that provides the child's return to the school program must assess the child's needs for transitional service and make appropriate services available. One positive effect of Public Law 94-142 on educational services for children who have been served in a hospital setting by special education is that the removal of the child from such a program or a change of the child's placement (return to the home school) must be accomplished through the ARD Committee. This will allow for continuous monitoring of the child's progress as she moves from one setting to the other. Likewise, the handicapped child who has remained in the classroom is assured of continued efforts at maintaining her integration in the classroom.

CHAPTER 6

The Reality in Psychosocial Focus

THOMAS A. HOLLAND
KATY MAXWELL
DONNA COPELAND
ALLISON STOVALL

The discussion of psychosocial issues of the "reality" took a variety of turns according to the concerns of those who spoke. To approach psychological and social aspects of persons (children and their families) involved in reintegration implies indeed a multiplicity of concerns and dimensions.

Included in the discussion were themes of support for families and the need for adequate transmission of information. Support matters were examined as needs for counseling for family members of cancer patients, both in medical and in school settings by appropriate personnel. The topic of transmitting information adequately—an enormous task—generated input and queries from medical, school, and parent attendees. Intended and unintended meanings, both spoken and written, are part of the complex task of sending and receiving needed data. A sense of the need for collaboration in this regard and a willingness to try seemed engendered by the participants' dialogue. One example, the use of labels in schools and in the hospital, as well as the implications of the labels for all persons concerned, was addressed at length.

Public Law 94-142 has had many positive effects on handicapped students and their families. It has also produced some unforeseen negative effects in both families and schools because of the sometimes unrealistic expectations it has generated. The law *seems* to promise to parents (although it does not *actually* promise) that each handicapped child will receive not just an appropriate education, but rather a perfect education—a perfect teacher, classroom, and peers, unlimited related services, absolutely the best individualized programs, etc., etc. The schools, no doubt, would be delighted to provide a perfect education, but a number of thorny realities limit their ability to "deliver." Funds are limited and as a result, districts have difficulty in providing the amounts of related services, which parents might consider optimal services, such as speech therapy, physical therapy, occupational therapy, vocational training, and counseling. Teachers and administrators must contend with the ocean of paperwork required to comply with the law. This can take time and energy away from the process of education itself and wear on the enthusiasm of special educators. Schools need to be honest with parents and present a realistic picture of what can and cannot be provided. Understanding the limitations of the schools puts dissatisfied parents in a position to constructively assist the schools, for example, by advocating increased tax revenues.

Public Law 94-142 guarantees that a handicapped child be educated in the "least restrictive environment"—that each child be mainstreamed to the extent that he or she can benefit. The concept of mainstreaming has much in it to recommend; it "normalizes" the handicapped child's experience and also prepares the child for the realities of living in a "normal" world. However, actually implementing the worthy intent of the law has unveiled a variety of problems. The law seems to imply that all teachers are capable of and interested in accommodating handicapped children in their classes, but this is not necessarily so for all teachers. Some teachers resent the addition of a handicapped student to their class, and yet they may be considered excellent teachers. Additionally, mainstreaming can be purely cosmetic, when it is done more to comply with the law than to benefit the child. To meet the intent of the law, considerable preparation is needed. Teachers need more training about the needs of handicapped students and techniques of accommodating them in "normal" classrooms so that they will not feel frightened, unprepared, or imposed upon. Also important is the need for preparing the "normal" students in classrooms and schools where handicapped children are mainstreamed. If these children have some understanding of the causes of handicaps and particularly of the experience of what it is like to be handicapped, they are often more accepting and mainstreaming is more beneficial for everyone.

Public Law 94-142 mandates that a child's parents be included in the educational planning for their child. This aspect of the law has spawned frustration for both the parents and the schools. Many parents respond with an enthusiasm to be included that makes some in the schools feel uncomfortable. Because the law has produced unrealistic expectations for many parents, educators may feel threatened by a parent's eagerness to be included and such educators may react defensively or uncooperatively, thus frustrating parents.

Clear and honest communication can do much to dispel the adversary relationship that has sometimes divided parent and school, as can the continued awareness that they share the common goal to serve the child. Interestingly, the law has resulted in some frustration with a lack of parental involvement for the schools as well as with perceived "over" involvement. Since the law mandates that parents be included in planning and efforts are made to encourage parental attendance at planned meetings, there is frustration among educators when parents seem uninterested and do not attend or inquire about the planning. Again, improved communication may benefit the situation by dispelling any parental fears about the meeting and making clear the value of parents' ideas and the "team effort" required to effectively educate the handicapped.

Public Law 94-142 has the potential to revolutionize in a very positive way the relationship of families, schools, and the medical profession in serving the educational needs of handicapped children. For this potential to be realized, it is essential that efforts be made to open the lines of communication among those three spheres. The strengths and limitations of each must be openly and honestly shared so that the expectations generated by the law can be attainable rather than impossible. As this communication begins to occur, the frustrations currently generated by the law can be minimized and a real partnership forged. The discussion groups, in fact, served to realize this goal to some extent.

Points of discussion centered around a number of psychosocial areas: 1) awareness, 2) communication, 3) attitudes, 4) expectations, and 5) training and education.

A sense of heightened *awareness* of the problem and need for action were apparent in the group discussion, and this increasing awareness seems to be reflective of that which is growing in the general public, and which perhaps received its first impetus from Public Law 94-142. There is still apathy in the community, but now the schools and parents seem to be saying, "How do we approach one another effectively?" There was general agreement that a realistic approach was more sensible, that is, rather than attempting to effect major changes in society, possibilities should be discussed given the society and the school system as they are.

Thus, the need for better *communication,* particularly between the parents and the schools, was consistently expressed. Parents of medically exceptional children need to be closely involved, and they need to be counseled about what they can realistically expect from the school and from their child. There needs to be better clarification about the possibilities for the child. One problem in communication has to do with the differing points of view between parents and school officials. The latter is often based on theoretical knowledge, while the former could be seen as more practical knowledge coming from experience. Friction seems to arise out of the tension between these two approaches, which results in some degree of defensiveness in the initial dialogues.

First and foremost, prevailing *attitudes* toward exceptional children should be addressed. For instance, there are teachers who view the admission of an exceptional child to their classroom as a flaw in perfection. They are sometimes intimidated by medical aspects of the child's life, and the psychological effect of obvious impairment may be one of threat to the teacher's own sense of effectiveness and perfection.

Teacher's attitudes and defensiveness are only one element in the matrix; detrimental attitudes of the parents may also interfere with reintegration. For instance, parents may at times attempt to deny the reality of their child's limitations and insist that others act as if they do not exist. One demonstration of this attitude is found in parents who impede cooperation between the medical community and schools by instructing the hospital not to inform the school of their child's psychiatric hospitalization. Thus, attitudes of shame and intolerance for differences may obstruct the effective reintegration of the child.

Expectations of others range from wanting the school to provide complete care with no involvement on the part of the parents to the parents wanting to provide complete schooling at home. There is a need to state what parents and schools can realistically expect of one another, given the constraints of limited funds and personnel. Very important in this respect are the interchanges between parents and schools that frankly state what each side expects of the other.

Finally, there is clearly a need to *train* and *educate* teachers about students requiring special educational considerations. This training should include not only information on the technical aspects of care, but also some exploration and insight into attitudes and feelings toward special or "imperfect" children.

In brief, significant problems exist in integrating the medically exceptional child into the school system. It was agreed that defensiveness on the part of parents and school personnel in dealing with these problems interferes with communication and thus impedes the effective achievement of the goal. One decisive action that has served to open up the dialogue and to encourage better communication has been The Education for All Handicapped Children Act of 1975 (Public Law 94-142).

CHAPTER 7

Psychosocial Factors in Reintegration

ALLISON STOVALL
THOMAS A. HOLLAND
KATY MAXWELL
DONNA R. COPELAND

This group discussion centered on psychosocial factors in the reintegration of the medically exceptional child. The issue of labeling was the focus. Several times allusions were made to Dr. Bartholome's point that health care providers create labels for patients. These labels, terms that emphasize different needs or lend themselves to stereotyping, can be barriers to assimilating the student into the school environment. When labels are overemphasized, children and their families experience the discomfort of enforced social distance, though the enforcement may be subtle. School personnel, despite specialized training, may create this distance as a result of the anxiety attached to their perception of these labels. This may impede their ability to help the classmates of the patient/student to accept him as an individual unencumbered by labels.

Fostering reintegration is dependent on an educational process that uses labels or informational tools rather than obstacles to understanding. With the passage of Public Law 94-142, there has been increased emphasis on helping the medically exceptional child. The educational community has to bear in mind the impact of these children on the children with no special medical needs.

These two student populations have been isolated from one another to a large degree until the implementation of this law. Educational professionals need to teach their students, by information and example, how to accept those children who have been labeled. It is important in the process to defuse the stigma that may be attached to the labels carried by patient/students.

School personnel need to be educated by health care providers regarding the special needs of the medically exceptional child if reintegration is to succeed. This need was clearly stated by members of different disciplines within the educational community.

Several vehicles for providing information to educators were discussed. School counselors were eager to know what methods the medical community used for helping parents. If parents are assisted cognitively and emotionally, they can enhance the adaptation of their children in resuming their place in school. They can also serve as liaisons between hospital and school as providers of information. Representatives of the hospital assured them that parental adaptation was viewed as critical to the adaptation of the child. To this end, counseling groups were considered. It was thought helpful to provide them with comprehensive data on the child's diagnosis, treatment, and capabilities for normal activity. Recognition of the importance of the parent's role is inherent in family-centered care.

Repeatedly, school personnel requested that medical personnel provide them with information on the patient's disease and his adaptation to disease and treatment. Ideally, in the view of educational professionals, medical personnel could give them a psychological profile or a written report from the various health care disciplines. This would be analogous to the written discharge plan that goes to a home care agency when such a referral is made. At the very least, the school personnel felt it would be helpful for the hospital to provide the school with a name to contact.

Currently, the hospital-based teacher takes the responsibility for communicating with the children's schools routinely, while physician and mental health professionals do so only as the need arises in exceptional situations. It was clear from the discussion that school personnel felt the need for medical and psychosocial data as well as educational data. As pointed out in the course of the discussion, medical professionals are at risk of reinforcing the labeling process when they provide written material of the kind requested. The format and content of such a report would have to guard against excessive labeling.

This discussion provided a forum for interchange among educational and health care professionals on issues of mutual concern. Those in pediatrics learned of the hunger that exists in the educational field for special knowledge of the needs of their patients. It was clear that many held the view that the medical community carries a major responsibility for educating patients, parents, and the public in this way. In pushing this point, one elementary counselor questioned why physicians place so much responsibility with the schools. A pediatrician pointed out that children in chronic treatment spend far more time in school than in the hospital, making schools primary areas for socialization.

The discussion clearly bore out Dr. Bartholome's contention that stretching the concept of the normally sick child beyond the therapeutic environment into the community is very difficult.

Section III
THE PROBLEM

Introduction

DONNA R. COPELAND

When first thinking about this introduction and what The Problem of reintegrating the medically exceptional child involves, my thoughts focused on the word provide. Being able to provide the opportunity for an appropriate education in the proper setting for each child is, broadly speaking, the first part of the problem.

The second part of the problem is related to the concept of reciprocity, which holds in all human relationships. Not only must we provide, but the child and parents must be able and willing to take advantage of the opportunities offered.

At present, there are a number of hindrances standing in the way of successfully meeting both of these aspects of the problem when a child is chronically or periodically ill. In terms of the individual child and his family, a certain degree of willingness for the child to go to school is first and foremost. The family must consider school important. Perhaps surprisingly, not only the child but also the parents may be ambivalent about schooling. The mother may feel that no one can take care of her child as well as she. The child may have lost confidence in his ability to perform and interact with others during a long course of illness and treatment. The mother may find she has devoted so much time to her sick child that other relationships and duties have slipped in importance and that, furthermore, she is curiously dependent on her child to provide *her* with a sense of mastery and accomplishment and being needed. If her son goes to school, whatever will she do?

However much these types of problems are valid, according to a study by the Spinettas (1), a greater share of the problem lies in how to accommodate and assimilate into the school system: A child who has been absent and thus requires extra help to catch up; A child who is "disruptive" in the sense of stirring up questions and feelings in others about human frailty and vulnerability; And a child who may have incurred side effects from the illness and treatment that have affected the ability to learn, to concentrate, to remember, or to use the senses.

In considering the statement that all are created equal, one can make an error in interpreting this to mean that in providing for others, standardized care and treatment is all that is required. That is if we provide a certain set of circumstances and let all help themselves; that is sufficient. We now realize, however, that equal rights and equal abilities and chances are not the same. Because individual needs vary, providing equal changes means doing different things for different people. Our greatest challenge is to decide how we can best assure an atmosphere of spontaneity, encouragement, and satisfaction in achievement for *all* our children. To meet this challenge may require first expanding our notions of what is *acceptable* to be, and then deciding what different kinds of children require for a healthy learning environment, one that encourages the child toward achieving the goals of maturation and growth.

Mrs. Catherine van Eys, a teacher in the Regional Day School Program for the Deaf in the Houston Independent School District, will discuss the many problems with which schools are confronted in resocializing not just the handicapped but all children. Mrs. van Eys is well qualified to speak on this subject as evidenced by her many certifications to teach children who are multiply and orthopedically handicapped, as well as those who are deaf. She received a B.A. degree from Vanderbilt University and an M.A. degree from George Peabody College.

Parents are an excellent source of information about the needs of their own children, and Mr. Wright and Mrs. Warco are representative of those interested and willing to collaborate with the schools in educational goals for their children. They will be approaching the problem from two very different kinds of experiences in getting educational help for their children. Both will be stressing a theme common to this conference, that of the necessity for flexibility in meeting the needs of different types of children.

Mr. Jim Wright, a graduate of the University of California at Berkeley, is presently in the field of computing as a senior staff systems analyst at Shell Oil Company. Mr. and Mrs. Wright have several children who have needed special learning environments, and he has some pertinent comments to make about mainstreaming and classroom atmosphere, pointing out how there are still problems in these areas that need our attention.

Mrs. Judy Warco, a graduate of the University of Houston, is a certified teacher; she will address the problem from the point of view of both parent and school system. She and her husband have a sense of cooperation with the school system in providing for the special needs of their son and she sees this kind of cooperation as a key factor in achieving positive results.

Dr. Albert Gunn, who will discuss The Hidden Handicap, is both a lawyer and a physician. He studied law in New York and later studied medicine in Ireland at the National University. He initially qualified in medicine at the Royal College of Physicians and the Royal College of Surgeons of England. Doctor Gunn is an internist by specialty and a Fellow of the American College of Physicians. His interest in the area of handicaps is longstanding, as shown by his work as a consultant to the White House Conference on Handicapped Individuals. Presently, he has a number of roles, but principally he is Assistant Director (Hospitals) and Associate Professor of Medicine at The University of Texas System Cancer Center.

REFERENCES

1. Spinetta, J. J. and Deasy-Spinetta, P.: Living with Childhood Cancer. St. Louis: C. V. Mosby, Publishers, 1981.

CHAPTER 8

School as the Arena for Resocialization

CATHERINE VAN EYS

The decade of the eighties will be an exciting and interesting time for the teaching profession. While many changes in education began to take place following World War II, the pace of these changes accelerated through the sixties and seventies and from those changes emerged the belief that the schools affect the welfare of our country and that ignorance is a handicap this nation cannot afford. Schools set children free to develop their natural ability, and thus they will preserve, it is hoped, the ideals established by our forefathers of liberty, justice, and equality for all. But while the classical ideal of school is represented by that statement, in current practice that often translates in a use of schools that is very different from traditional teaching of knowledge and values. This paper will describe the change in expectations parents and society have of the schools.

The reflections in this paper come from personal experiences. My teaching career began in the early fifties and continues until now. The concept of "school" that was taught in my home is different from the one generally heard in conversations with parents and children today. Often one hears parents excuse the fact that their child did not do assigned homework because he was involved in a sports activity. My father believed school prepared one for college to be able to participate in the fullness of life. One studied Latin diligently to improve one's vocabulary and to learn logical thinking. A profession would evolve from this education, but was not the only purpose. None of this discussion was "if" you attend school, do well, and attend college, but "when." Parents would have been surprised at the suggestion that school was the place for socialization or resocialization. Yet, currently the school is the arena in which socialization is expected to take place. To discuss this it is well at this point to define exactly what the phrase "socialization" means and how the word is defined—for all of us have a definition that reflects past experiences and knowledge. The verb "socialize" is defined as: "to adapt or convert to the needs of a social group" (1). The definition given for "school" is: "any institution devoted primarily to imparting knowledge or to develop certain skills or talents, especially an educational institution for children" (1). Colleges and universities were therefore included in the definition, but the emphasis of the concept "school" was on children. When the definitions of socialization and school are combined, one has a statement that says: a school is a place for children to be taught knowledge or to develop skills and talents that would meet the needs of a social group. To evaluate whether this concept of socialization fits the new ideas of the sixties and seventies we should review our recent history.

World War II had awakened many people. Many left home and travelled (some abroad) for the first time. The depression was over. New hope surfaced as people moved into the 1950s. Frequently one reads that in the past the schools and teachers did a poor job and discriminated against many. Certainly, studies in the 1950s show that many school districts had exceedingly poor facilities available for both white and black children (2). Unless one was fortunate to live in an area where schools were well funded, most education was of poor quality. Yet, as a beginning teacher in an inner city school, I observed teachers who did far more than present academic material to a child. They did not dismiss the home and all its problems. Those teachers worked long and hard to aid entire families to share in the "Great American Dream"—The Dream that armed with skills learned in school (reading, writing, and arithmetic) one could better one's self and partake of the opportunities presented here in America. This belief and desire were frequently talked about when parents and teachers interacted—whether in the school or in the home. Personal and home problems of a wide variety were presented to the teachers by the parents with the sure knowledge that aid of some measure would be forthcoming.

In this period the philosophy of the parents seemed to be to teach the children skills to further them in the job market and self-help skills to make life more comfortable. Even our poorest parents maintained that discipline was necessary for a child to learn in a classroom. They shouldered their part of the responsibility to aid the school. There are, of course, always exceptions one could cite, but exceptions should not be used to illustrate a point. Many of these parents represented a group of people who lived a lifestyle that was foreign to me. I had never known adults who were unable to read or write.

During these years teachers heard little discussion of parents suing either teachers or schools. Many teachers aided families in ways that now one would hesitate to even consider: planning funerals and taking a child to the hospital for care. Perhaps the parents' lack of skills made them more aware of the importance of learning. In my second year, I was placed in a school that drew students from a higher socioeconomic level, but was still lower middle class. Again the same philosophy prevailed. Children had good attendance records and parents were in and out of the school daily to aid the teachers. As a result there was excellent discipline throughout the school. A follow-up survey of this group of third graders (approximately 30) indicates a majority finished high school and four entered college.

By the mid-1950s tremendous changes were taking place in America, conceptually, intellectually, and concretely. The landmark decision *Brown* v. *Board of Education,* Topeka, Kansas, 1954, which was reviewed as the representative desegregation court case by the Supreme Court, stated that dual school systems

were no longer permitted (3). Henceforth schools would be integrated. Later, even more important, *de facto* segregation became
outlawed (4). One almost needs to have been on the scene to
appreciate some of the problems schools faced. The court had
decreed what is to be. Many segments of society agreed. An equally large segment of the population disagreed. The school was left
to implement the decision. If changes in thinking are to be
effected, introducing new ideas to children is a positive way of
approaching the problem; adults are much more difficult to
change, witness the energy crisis. In Nashville, Tennessee, the plan
was to integrate one grade a year in the neighborhood schools.
Initially, this was rather successful. With the parents in close
proximity, conferences could be held to solve problems before
they became serious. When children study, play, and eat together,
it is difficult for any group in society to maintain old beliefs about
another culture.

After an interlude of raising a family, I returned to an inner city
school with the assignment to teach mentally retarded children.
This school had all the problems in actuality that could be listed,
particularly integration. However, the teachers accepted the
challenge of integration and did, in fact, a remarkable job. It was
an older group of teachers and I often wonder if their age and
experience were the reasons for the stability of the school. Many
of the adults in the neighborhood and community did not show
the same calm approach. It was the year of sit-ins and school
house burnings. Yet today, changes from that time are too numerous to list and a large percentage of people know no other way.
If you were to ask whether a complete socialization of minority
groups has taken place, many would say no, while others would
say that we've come a long way. It is an ongoing process in our
society.

Now we have a new definition of minorities to consider. As the
fifties merged into the sixties, several ideas were surfacing. Integration marched steadily forward in all arenas of life. In the 1960s,
child advocates became vocal. They were often needed for the

benefit of the child. Simultaneously, exciting new breakthroughs were made in knowledge in many different fields of study because of liberal federal funding of biomedical research. A new family came on the American scene with a tremendous impact, in the person of John F. Kennedy. Almost immediately the American people learned about the mentally retarded sister, Rosemary. Here was a prominent family that openly acknowledged a retarded member. In numerous articles her life story was told. It was written how she was educated. People were told how the decision was made to place Rosemary in a special home. This was not the usual behavior of families in the higher socioeconomic classes who had a retarded family member. In the classrooms of the educable mentally retarded, one might find several children from a lower socioeconomic family with no stigma attached. However, in our classes for severely retarded, the wealthier parents were often embarrassed or at least misunderstood by the general public when seen with their child. So often the appearance of the child or his behavior gave clues to the severe retardation. It was a relief to have the Kennedy family bring mental retardation "out of the closet." By their impetus, funding for child development research from the Kennedy Foundation and the federal government became available. A Kennedy Center was established on the Peabody Campus. It strongly influenced teacher training, graduate studies, and the public school system. The Kennedy Center generated action in all areas of exceptionality and handicaps, so that a most exciting group of professors were gathered under the remarkable chairmanship of Lloyd Dunn (best known for the Peabody Picture Vocabulary Test and Peabody Kits). Persons such as Lloyd Dunn were teaching new ideas in dealing with the handicapped to undergraduate and graduate students in a variety of fields. It was Lloyd Dunn's electrifying speech in 1967 that rocked the educational world. He stated that mainstreaming handicapped children was the answer rather than self-contained classrooms (5). His contention was that children would fare better academically, which was still one of our basic criteria. During this period new ideas began to be discussed about the advisability of placing children in institutions versus home settings. Questions were asked about the impact of stimulation versus nonstimulation. Determinations of the learning rate of a child were considered.

At the same time that these ideas were exploding, a new phenomenon was occurring that was dividing the American people with new beliefs emerging in the younger age group concerning the meaning of life. The drug culture was born. Extreme views were expressed concerning the Vietnam War. The conscientious objector was a new type of young adult. Many young people dropped out of life on drugs. Schools were suddenly faced with increased problems of such children on drugs. Little parental support was given because parents were equally lost and bewildered. I have no idea how the drug problem was dealt with elsewhere in the mid-1960s, but in Seattle, where I was teaching, drugs were easily obtainable in the high schools. By the late 1960s even elementary schools faced these problems. Again school personnel were attempting to meet the needs of the community with little or no training for the task.

On this point I must digress a moment. My educational training began in the late 1940s and through the intervening years I have continued to take courses in different areas. As knowledge has been acquired about certain handicaps, that information has been taught. In cases of retardation we know much more about Down's Syndrome. In deafness and blindness, new syndromes have been identified and described. Children with emotional problems and learning disabilities are better understood. In regular school we have moved through the era of "new math" and the new "transformational" grammar of Chomsky with his new linguistics and deep structures, which has been the new direction in the subject of English. Yet, teacher training has not changed basically. The basic courses still remain, theory of education, history of the state, and core courses, but few courses are offered in the psychosocial aspects of school as society now perceives the school. Now with the advent of Public Law 94-142, teachers receive a general course in special education to prepare them to meet the needs of children who might be placed in their classroom. So it is no wonder that many teachers feel uncertain about receiving these children. Also many of the older teachers have not even had the one course in special education. It is imperative that we acknowledge that this public law has caused changes and find a solution that does not involve the teacher staying after school for inservice courses that simply list the problems with simplistic answers. Industry would not attempt to retrain its personnel in such a fashion. Added to the difficulty imposed by myriad teaching styles, teachers are faced with an incredible amount of paperwork, particularly in special education. This is compounded by the low pay in comparison to cost of training and alternative job opportunities.

Public Law 94-142 is one of the major changes to happen in the 1970s. This law states that "All children are entitled to an education in the least restrictive environment." (6) I suspect that few people anticipated the impact that this simple statement would have upon our society. It was true that many parents who had handicapped children had met with less than enthusiastic support from school officials when they had attempted to find placement for their children. Sometimes the reasons given by school administrators were correct, there simply was no program designed or even feasible to meet the needs of only one or two children. Even if such programs existed, in rural counties and smaller towns they were less well funded compared with the metropolitan areas. However, one is often left with the impression that little concern was expressed by the school officials. Consequently, parent groups banded together and insisted as taxpayers that programs should be designed to meet the needs of their children. Once Public Law 94-142 became a reality, those same school officials who previously offered no hope, suddenly began to discover available options to avoid being sued. Do not misinterpret these remarks. All through the 1960s, many large urban districts had designed programs for these children. In most instances such districts have not had as many problems. The smaller districts were the ones in most difficulty. To use an analogy, it simply is not possible to have in each county in Texas the same facilities that M. D. Anderson Hospital does. Not only is it not practical, it would not even be rational.

A large majority of the children not previously served have been children located through "Child Find." They are often children who have multiple handicaps. These children are frequently severely retarded and require a tremendous amount of personnel to meet even everyday needs. In this day of rising costs and income threats to schools, such as California's Proposition 13, school officials are faced with the problem of the loaves and the fishes without faith of miraculous sufficiency. It is a major question where adequate financing is to come from and how the available funds can be equitably divided among all children. In the fall of 1979 a case was filed against a school district to require a teacher or nurse to daily catheterize a child at school (7). This would require several members of the staff to be trained in this procedure because no one has a 100 percent attendance record. As reported in the January 14, 1980, *Houston Post,* a suit was filed against the Galveston Independent School District to provide temporary care for a 16-year-old boy at a private residential-care facility until the Alvin School District develops an appropriate program for this youth. Furthermore, for having failed so far to do this, $500,000 for damages were sought. These types of cases certainly generate monstrous problems for administrators to solve. These cases also raise issues concerning the obligations of the schools to children.

Looking at children with a chronic illness such as cancer, one must remember that this is another new problem. Prior to 1970, the median life span of a child with lymphocytic leukemia was a matter of months. Now in 1980, more than half of all children with this disease live indefinitely. Consider the group of all cancer children, and look at some of their problems that will surface during remission when they are returning to school (8). The list would include drug-induced loss of hair, amputation of a limb, a visible tumor—in short, problems that affect the self-image of a child. Coupled with the visible problems are the emotional difficulties. Many teachers substitute pity for acceptance of any handicap. In that way they convey to the student that it is acceptable not to do well in school. After all, "*you* have cancer." They may even be implying death is around the corner. And usually the home school teacher is given little if any assistance by medical personnel. This leaves the teachers very insecure, not knowing if precautions should be taken and if so what. They do not know what they should do if the child complains of feeling poorly. If the chronically ill child goes out of remission, the school teacher in the home school is expected to cooperate with the hospital teacher for the child to have a smooth, uninterrupted educational program. This requires good communication among all parties, which can be very difficult.

The problems of the home teacher are massive compared with the hospital teacher. The hospital teacher is on the scene—she can ask questions of the physicians, nurses, and mental health workers. She will come to know family members. None of this is available for the home school teacher. It is easy for the medical profession to lose sight of the loneliness one can feel when these responsibilities are given to you.

In recounting changes through the years, one thing becomes clear. Schools are not static institutions, but are continually changing to meet the needs of society. As changes in customs, in thinking, and in the economic realities take place in the world, the school is used as a tool to mold children to a new way of thinking. One of the major difficulties in the desegregation of schools was challenging the white Anglo-Saxon Protestant beliefs that had been handed down carefully from parent to child. In the school setting, children are able to see the fallacy of this thinking. We are currently facing cultural differences with the massive immigration of foreign born. How shall we educate these groups as Americans, leaving intact their identities?

The question before us then is what is the role of the school: Is the school the arena for socialization? The answer based on history and experience tends to be: Yes, as thoughts and ideas in society change, the schools are used to teach these new beliefs.

Teachers who stay in the profession must be flexible in their thinking and constantly expose themselves to continuing education through lectures, workshops, and readings to learn as much as possible about society's problems, for those are the problems that will surface tomorrow in the schools. Now that the problem of the chronically ill child has surfaced, teachers should be supported in the role of resocialization for the medically exceptional child with whom they have been entrusted.

REFERENCES

1. Funk and Wagnalls Standard Desk Dictionary. New York, 1974.
2. Brickman, S. S., Lehrer, S., eds. Education and the Many Faces of the Disadvantages: Cultural and Historical Perspectives. New York: John Wiley and Sons, 1972.
3. Lapali, A. D. *Brown* vs. *Board of Education,* 347, U.S. 483 (1954). Education and the Federal Government. New York: Mason Chamber Publishers, 1975.
4. *Hobson* v. *Hansen,* U.S. District Court for the District of Columbia. Congressional Record 113, No. 98, June 21, 1967, H. 7655–7700.
5. Dunn. L. M. Special education for the mildly retarded—Is much of it justified? Except. Child., 35:5–22, 1968.
6. Education for All Handicapped Children Act of 1975. Public Law 94-142, 29 Nov. 1975, 89 STAT. 773–96: Federal Register 42(163):42474–518, 23 Aug. 1977.
7. *Henry and Mary T.* v. *the State of Texas,* Filed in the U.S. District Court, Northern Division of Texas, Dallas. Patrick E. Higginbotham presiding.
8. Kirten, C., Liverman, M. Special educational needs of the child with cancer. J. Sch. Health, 47:170–173, 1977.

CHAPTER 9

The Teacher as Parent, the Parent as Teacher — One Special Case

JUDY WARCO

The weeks preceding Thanksgiving this past November will long be remembered by myself and my family. I had just agreed to replace a teacher after Thanksgiving until she could return following surgery, and, less than two weeks later, I found a small hard knot in the calf of my younger son's leg. That was on November 16, 1979, and by December 5, our quiet, happy, secure life had come to an abrupt end.

Realizing that what I had found might be malignant, my first action was to go to our family physician. He then referred us to an orthopedist, and at this point, I met with school officials to advise them of the very real possibility of my not being able to fulfill the commitment made to teach. Even at this stage, total cooperation of the school was attained.

On November 30, a diagnosis of Ewing's sarcoma was made and confirmed by a bone biopsy. Before explaining the subsequent proceedings, I would like to give a brief view of our family before cancer entered our lives.

My husband and I are both college graduates with his degree being in engineering and mine in special education for the blind and visually handicapped and in elementary education. We have two sons, Laurance, age 8, and Daniel, age 6. Laurance is very bright, inquisitive, and outgoing. Daniel, the younger, is also very bright, but very shy and quiet, quite the opposite of Laurance.

Prior to his illness, Daniel attended school regularly and was one of the top children in his class; but being a quiet child, he enjoyed doing things by himself. He was a sensitive child, wanting to please those around him. He was secure and well adjusted. Although he was quiet and shy, he made friends easily and was well liked by his classmates.

Now let me return to our life after the initial diagnosis. From Thanksgiving to Christmas, Daniel's education became of secondary importance to us. Daniel was pulled from his classroom for massive testing, for the beginning of chemotherapy, and for unexpected hospitalization as a result of the chemotherapy. He attended school only five days during that 30-day period of time. To his teacher fell the uneasy task of trying to explain to his worried classmates what was happening to Daniel, why he was on crutches, why he couldn't come to school, why he had lost all of his hair. Laurance's teacher had to explain the same things and also had to help Laurance adjust to the enormous changes in his life as a result of his brother's illness.

While Laurance's world remained somewhat stable, Daniel's world became filled with strangers—strangers who wanted to take pictures of his body, strangers who wanted to know what he was thinking, strangers who wanted his blood, and little strangers who were in varying stages of baldness or who were missing limbs or who had funny red lines drawn on their faces and bodies. After much contemplation, my husband and I decided to try to make life as near normal as possible in an effort to eliminate some of the strangers and regain some control over our child's destiny, even if that control was very little.

By now the realization of the lengthy duration of the treatment began to dawn in our lives and once again education was becoming a prime concern. Because Daniel's life had been so full of chaos and strangers, we decided to approach the school district with what my husband and I felt would be the most satisfactory solution: Not to enroll in the homebound program, but rather work with his teacher and allow me to teach him at home under her directions.

When we first approached the school, we felt that asking for their help, rather than demanding their help, would yield the results we sought. Daniel's teacher had already demonstrated interest and concern by "educating" his classmates about our dilemma. We approached her with the following plan: First, Mrs. Smith would continue to grade and assign Daniel's work. Second, I would be given teacher's manuals and proceed under her directions. And third, our other son, Laurance, in an effort to involve him as much as possible, would be the liaison carrying work to and from school.

Upon her approval of the plan, we then approached the principals involved and their approval was given. At every point of decision making, the school cooperated. Notes were sent home explaining the danger of being exposed to chicken pox so parents and teachers kept the school nurse informed. Class visitations were permitted to keep Daniel in touch with his classmates. Other classes within the school sent get well wishes. And the school counselor provided answers for questions we had concerning Daniel's well being both educationally and mentally.

Without the total cooperation of this team of educators, Daniel's educational well being would have deteriorated drastically. By allowing this type of educational process, whereby his original teacher maintained control, Daniel felt an integral part of his school. No matter how long he was absent, he knew that his desk was still there awaiting his return and that his classmates would still accept him, hair or no hair. Their initial reaction upon seeing him bald for the first time was proof of his teacher's excellent preparations; they hugged him and clapped upon his return. No homebound program could have ever provided this total feeling of acceptance.

Having mother for a teacher presented problems at first. There was resistance at each attempt initially until Daniel realized there was no other alternative. A daily schedule was established and the program was begun. The first objective was to catch up for the past month's work and go ahead as surgery was pending and we knew more hospitalization would be necessary. Work was sent for grading and the first report card was sent home just like all the other children. Teaching on a one-to-one basis affords many more opportunities for subject expansion. As an example, we baked chocolate chip cookies for our culminating lesson in science on the five senses. We planted flowers and tomatoes and put them under a grow light for another unit.

In February, surgery was scheduled and performed, and while awaiting the surgery, Daniel chose his subject for his science fair project. Daniel wrote for his project the following:

> Cancer is a bad disease. It may kill you. I had to go to the hospital. They put me in surgery for a bone biopsy. The scariest test was when they X-rayed all my bones because I was left in a room all by myself. The machines are big, but they don't hurt you. I get chemotherapy treatments now. When I get them I feel scary. They make me sick sometimes. My hair came out too and it hurt when it came out. Some people have cancer like me. They have to go to the hospital like me. I feel bad about having cancer. When I don't have cancer, I don't feel bad. I don't know why I have cancer, and nobody knows why except God. When I grow up I want to be a doctor at M. D. Anderson and find out why people have cancer.

In our opinion, Daniel's project was the combination of many people's efforts—his physicians, his teachers, his peers, his family. It demonstrated that although we had not asked for this chronic illness—and that is what we consider cancer to be—we had it, and most important, had accepted the reality of it.

My topic has been what I, as a parent, expected from the school. I guess that while I took actions to achieve what I wanted, I never really examined the underlying reasons for those actions until now. I expected the school, rather I expected the school personnel involved, to provide a stable educational environment in an otherwise chaotic envirionment, to make my medically exceptional child less exceptional, to help my child accept the reality of his environment, and, in return, to have the educational environment accept him. But most of all, I wanted the school and the children to love and accept the new Daniel as they had the old Daniel and my expectations and wants have been fulfilled beyond my wildest dreams.

Although we neither reside in nor attend the Houston Independent School District, I firmly believe that any parent who is willing to work jointly with the school system, whether it be H.I.S.D. or the Clear Creek School District of which we are a part—whether the parents are certified teachers or not—can implement a program similar to the one we established. It has worked beautifully for us, but it has also required the extra work and cooperation of many dedicated educators. Being a former teacher, I know that teachers do care, but when there are 25 or more other students to educate, the parent must also care enough to do all that is possible in achieving the most feasible solution.

As an aftermath, Daniel returned to school on April 14, 1980, for a half day. It was his first day of attending school since December and he walked in, sat down, and resumed his place in the classroom. Although his attendance will be rather erratic in the next two years, his education will proceed without problems. The only problem I have now is that school lasts too long and now he has to miss "Battle of the Planets" each afternoon.

CHAPTER 10

Searching for More Understanding for the Child — Observations of a Parent

JIM WRIGHT

Our children, whether they be handicapped or not, need two things from education: one is a teacher and the other is a class. Parents want a teacher who wants to teach, who will not give up, and who respects our children. We need a teacher the students can respect. The class is necessary so that the children can have socialization. At times, it is tempting to keep the children at home and teach them ourselves, but that would leave out the class, the socialization, and leave their education incomplete.

To make the class functional, the teacher must be in control of the class. There must be discipline before learning can take place. A disabled child has a hard time learning when being ridiculed. An established norm of mutual respect and acceptance is what we would like to have in the class, in the community, and in the home. Sometimes the parents' expectations are not always met.

To appreciate what I am talking about, I will give a short health sketch and then an educational sketch of our daughter Cindy. Maybe then you will understand the context of our problem. Cindy is fourteen and a half years old and the fourth of six children. She had her first seizures when she was three months old. Since then she has had seizures most of her life, up until she was twelve and a half years old. And so seizures were something that had to be dealt with. Sometimes there were ten or twenty days during which there were no observable seizures, but then there would be day after day in which there would be one or two or a dozen seizures. This in itself is handicapping. She has further problems now because of the brain damage that resulted from the seizures. She has difficulty in speech and language development. She might also be classed as a cerebral palsied child because she does not have full motor control. And there are other problems too numerous to mention. These problems are not severe individually, but taken in total, they are a constant problem.

During December 1978, she had a severe headache; an evaluation, followed by brain surgery, revealed a malignant tumor. For that she has had radiation, with the resulting loss of hair. Now she is on chemotherapy with its problems. Yet she is still doing well.

Cindy's educational background is equally complex. We initially placed her in the Houston Speech and Hearing Center when she was about three years old to work on speech and language development. She was there when she normally might have started kindergarten, but then a change in the program of the center in the middle of that year left her without an adequate class. Therefore, we put Cindy into the local elementary school of the Houston Independent School District. It did not take long before the seizures scared the daylights out of her kindergarten teacher and we were informed by the school that Cindy would not be permitted to attend school more than one-half hour per day. Well, that was not very much. We then started with some testing through H.I.S.D. All this despite the fact that we had thoroughly informed the principal, the teacher, and the school nurse that Cindy had seizures and that there was not a lot they could do about it. We told them that she would be all right in a few minutes following the seizure. In fact, it was quite possible that they might not even notice all of the seizures. We spent the rest of that year testing and trying to put her into special educational classes, none of which worked out very well. We were not satisfied that all was being done to utilize fully her capabilities, so we enrolled her in a private school that she attended for six years. We were very happy with the results of that school, at least for four and a half years. But all schools have a problem. They are staffed with teachers, all of whom are human and not always able to deal with all problems. Cindy was once again finding that she had moved on to a teacher who could not deal with her problems. Consequently, her academic work started to suffer. The teachers at the private school did help Cindy to develop her gross motor skills, her academic skills, her social skills, and all the other skills a young child needs to learn. Cindy was doing very well until she reached a point where she was no longer developing academically.

Fortunately, by this time we had Public Law 94-142. Therefore, we felt that we now had a better opportunity to go back to H.I.S.D. and insist, as best we could, on their help to return her to the public schools. At that time, Cindy might have gone into the seventh grade, but we were afraid to put her into a large junior high school. Fortunately in the plan designed in the Admission Review and Dismissal Conference, and the resulting individualized educational program that was drawn up for her, she was allowed to have the option of going to an elementary school in our neighborhood. In fact, we lived between the elementary school and the junior high school, so that as far as distance went, they were both community schools. We decided on the elementary school, and this was where she started in September 1978. Educationally, that was a very good year. The school had a new principal and Cindy had a very understanding, very capable special education teacher who worked very well with her. Between the two of them and some mainstreaming into the regular sixth grade class, she was doing very well. The unfortunate circumstance is that was the year she had brain surgery. But that too turned out to be very fortunate in that the school was in the community. The other children in the classes, including her own brother who was in the sixth grade in the same school, understood her problems. The teacher and the principal were able to communicate with the students and teachers. Cindy was welcomed back to school as a kind of hero.

The following year she was ready to progress to the seventh grade. A basic problem within our school system, I believe, is the big gap in the move from the sixth grade in an elementary school to the seventh grade in a junior high school. There the students have a different teacher every hour. Therefore, there are many more teachers who must try to learn what Cindy's problems are, how to help her, how to keep her moving ahead. But I think Cindy regards this year as a fairly good year. She is very pushy about learning. She is very forward. She tries to be independent; she goes back and forth to school by herself, not with her brother. She belongs to a local AAU team and we no longer take her to and from her swimming exercises. She does all of these things very independently.

Cindy still, however, has a problem. Not all her teachers understand that she has some difficulty clearly understanding instructions. There is a communication problem at school. There is also a problem of discipline in such a large school with so many different teachers and so many different students for each teacher to handle. These are challenges that the school and the individual teachers must learn how to meet. We as parents certainly stand ready to explain our child's difficulty. We are willing to try to correct any behavioral problems that exist. But if we don't communicate, we can't get the job done. If we don't communicate, if the teacher does not accept and respect the child in the class, if the teacher really feels that this is one pupil you can ignore so that you will not have as much trouble, then we as parents have an insurmountable problem.

A great problem is the specialization of classes. We have major work classes, accelerated classes, regular classes, and special education classes. I could go on ad infinitum. Particularly in high school we see more and more segregation of classes. And all that I see left in the regular classes are what I would term the disabled and disinterested students. The disinterested student is one we do not quite understand yet. Perhaps you could call his the hidden problem. When you lump the disinterested and the disabled students together, you get a very difficult class for the teacher to handle. And it is a very difficult class for the disabled child to function in.

As I have said, I don't have the definitive solution, but we parents stand willing to work with the teachers. But it is sometimes difficult; few of us have their level of expertise, so our concerns aren't always clearly communicated. It seems too often the school is ready to switch you to another program rather than to refine the present program to make it work. Communication is the major element we lack. We may think we have a program designed to communicate with the teacher on a weekly basis. However, it always breaks down. Maybe after six weeks you hear that things haven't been doing very well. That is too late.

So my appeal to education is: give us good teachers, who are interested in teaching, who are not going to give up, and who are going to accept the child. Give us a class in which there is enough discipline where ridicule is held to a minimum, so that there is more understanding between students and between students and teachers.

CHAPTER 11

The Hidden Handicap

ALBERT GUNN

Handicap has a variety of meanings depending on circumstances, but is essentially a philosophical term. We often talk as if it were completely defined someplace, and indeed there are attempts at definitions contained in various laws. But ultimately, the word only has a meaning when you refer to a specific outcome. Toulouse-Lautrec and Søren Kierkegaard were handicapped in one sense, and yet who would not exchange places with them for their artistic and intellectual preeminence. The circumstances of a person's life govern whether some condition he has or doesn't have handicapped him. I would like to interject at this point the definition of "handicapped," realizing this may strike you as sophomoric.

> A race or any contest . . . in which in order to equalize chances of winning an artificial disadvantage is imposed on a supposedly superior contestant or an artificial advantage is given to one supposedly inferior. Also, an advantage given . . . or a disadvantage imposed. (1)

The second meaning is: figuratively, any advantage that renders success more difficult. (1)

My experience with the problem of analyzing the word "handicap" began when I was a health advisor and the designer of a set of criteria to employ handicapped people in a CETA Program. They were to be employed and given civil service tenure without reference to civil service examination and without going through many employment steps usually required in the particular county that was involved.

When you discuss handicaps from the standpoint of people who are looking for something like that, you will find a lot of people consider themselves handicapped in ways you never imagined. Your primary function is to prove that people are not handicapped. The circumstances governed the definition and its application.

This type of circumstantial definition has created a problem that has bedeviled the question of who is or who is not handicapped. On the one instance, many people do not want to be considered handicapped because it obstructs them and holds them back. They cannot get a certain job they like, e.g., a government commission driver's license. They do not want to be included among the handicapped. They can be enrolled in special programs, given pensions, or entitled to special treatment. The example already given of the CETA program covers this situation. Standing by itself the word handicap thus has no definite meaning and this has led to problems. On the other hand, there are people who would like to be considered handicapped because it entitles them to something.

In the past, most of the areas of handicap that have been discussed have concentrated on orthopedic conditions. In fact, isn't it true that when you think of a handicap, you think of people in wheelchairs or those with spinal cord injuries or other neurologic disorders? The association that most of us make is with problems with locomotion or the use of arms. This emphasis is due partly because the subjective handicap, one the handicapped person experiences but no one else can see, is often bound up with society's conception of malingers, goldbricks, and other perjorative terms of a like quality. Until recently when handicaps were discussed, the connotation was that the handicap could be seen and, more important, measured. If it couldn't be measured, then photographed or exactly categorized. It is easy to say a deaf person is handicapped because you can use an audiometer and precisely determine the extent of the handicap. Similarly, with a blind person there are charts and very exact definitions of just what constitutes blindness. But what about those conditions where nothing can be seen or measured. Society has been suspicious about this area. In some, the feeling has been that such handicaps were not worthy of our help or perhaps even our sympathy.

Dr. Bartholome (2) reviewed the recent development of the specialty of rehabilitation, or using its official name, Physical Medicine and Rehabilitation. Dr. Howard Rusk was the pioneer in the development of this medical specialty. He deserves tremendous credit. But I think it is very unfortunate that the term "physical medicine" should have been so prominently placed in the description of this medical specialty. Going further, I see the term "rehabilitation" as a very unfortunate term. The term I believe to be most appropriate to cover the process and goals we are discussing is *readaptation*. The word of rehabilitation brings to mind visions of dilapidated buildings or broken down cars. The problem is almost totally physical and our aim is to fix it up and get it going. Rehabilitation involves more of a static endeavor, wherein the artisan works on an object that remains passive or passively cooperative during the intervention. The reality with human beings is a dynamic process that may involve strengthening a limb or substituting one shell for another, but, most importantly and specifically, views the individual as a unit and as a whole. The process examines the individuals' relationships to their surroundings, whether these be the family, work place, or school. The fact that they recover 60% function of a limb tells us very little about their ability to live their life in a context that will make them happy.

In 1977, the White House Conference on Handicapped Individuals was held. It was attended by delegates from all over the United States. I had the privilege of being a delegate-at-large. I was an appointed and not an elected delegate. Elected delegates were drawn from the handicapped themselves and this was the proper method of selection. Who better than the handicapped know the needs and are able to design programs for the handicapped?

The providers of services and others working in the field were welcome as consultants, but were not given the role of decision makers. It was a good idea. The organizers did not want the conference dominated by providers, professionals, and bureaucrats. Those people were involved in designing services, getting grants, administering programs, or similar activities in relationship to the handicapped. They had the capacity to contribute, but properly were not the final decision makers.

During the course of the conference, I became aware of a movement that was spontaneously gathering force to propose a resolution on hidden handicaps. It was an interesting group of people joined in this endeavor. The spectrum of diseases represented were epilepsy, autism, communicative disorders, cystic fibrosis, diabetes, and neoplastic diseases, the last being my interest area. A resolution was framed to try to point up the real nature of certain types of handicaps, that unlike the orthopedic and similar disabilities that could not be seen but were no less real. The radical nature of this resolution was in making the disease a handicap itself. This was a new approach. A great deal of the conceptual groundwork for the resolution had been done by the mental health and mental retardation groups. They had raised the general level of consciousness and sensitivity to problems that caused handicaps and yet that had been considered "subjective" and not "objective."

There had been quite a change in the general appreciation of the public toward the mentally ill and retarded. This change involved considerable dedication and enthusiasm by many. The essential and underlying point had been made that every person is of worth and is entitled to just treatment by society. If we attempt to develop some persons to their full potential, we owe that to everyone. Whatever resources are required should be expended because all are equal before the law and entitled to equal treatment. The crucial point established was that because a person has a defect, he still is of value. Everyone could empathize with someone who had a missing limb. It could happen to anyone. But to regard schizophrenics as handicapped and not just as troublesome types who should be locked up was a real breakthrough. The hidden handicap was a logical progression of the line of thinking. The key building block of this progress has been the recognition of the absolute worth of every individual whether they are like everyone else or not.

One of the things about hidden handicaps that characterizes them and the treatment seen more with them is that they always disqualify persons from services or rights, but never serve as an entitlement. A person with epilepsy has trouble getting a driver's license, of becoming a swimming coach, and at one time couldn't even marry. But having epilepsy entitles the patient to no special treatment. Epileptics don't get a pension, nor are they considered disabled. To me this catch-22 like quality is the hallmark of the hidden handicap. A hidden handicap will keep you out of work, but won't let you receive unemployment compensation.

I once had the unpleasant duty of informing a young woman working in a District Attorney's office that she was fired because she had Hodgkin's disease. The medical examiner who had examined her had not disqualified her upon employment. Under the employment physical criteria, Hodgkin's disease was an absolute against employment irrespective of the stage of prognosis. The examining physician worked at the standards and certified her for employment anyway. You can imagine her reaction when she was told she could no longer be employed. It was very unfair. But it had the salutary effect of causing all of the medical standards then in effect for that organization to be scrapped. This was a happy ending in one case, but it is a sad commentary on the prevailing mentality that causes people to be fired for certain conditions and yet not be the recipients of special help because they are not "handicapped."

The problem in these areas is that there is suspicion by the public, the taxpayers, that we are trying to include people as handicapped who in some way play a role in their handicap. They are not tough, they don't "tough it out." They give up. They don't have fortitude. They are weak. This comes up time and again in these areas. Some people act as if the systemic effects of cancer are all in the mind. In fact, these misconceptions arose at the White House Conference on Handicapped Individuals because the people who did have standard types of disability, loss of limbs and various types of physical disorders, were leary of this resolution. They thought it would open a flood gate more or less to almost anyone claiming they were handicapped because they were tired or weak.

The conference was opened by President Carter and the Secretary of Health, Education, and Welfare, Califano. The Secretary had only recently been picketed at his office by a group of people in wheel chairs. This had raised awareness of the handicapped problems and Mr. Califano had recently signed regulations related to insuring rights for the handicapped. I think the demonstrations strengthened his hand in doing something he wanted to do. The public could vividly see the problems of the handicapped. But the persons who etched the images in the public mind were those with obvious problems. They were in wheel chairs or missing limbs. No one with Hodgkin's disease or a colostomy was prominent in all this. The President and the Secretary stated their general goal as bringing the handicapped to a position of parity with the rest of the American society. The atmosphere on the opening night was one of optimism and potential for advance. We had not come to the age of Proposition 13 and the era of dwindling resources yet.

The resolution was proposed from the floor after receiving the necessary signature. It was not on the original agenda. It was studied and then put to a vote after the conference ended. There were 393 votes for this resolution by the people present at the conference. There were only five resolutions out of all those considered that received more than 400 votes. One of those was a commendation to President Carter and another was a commendation to teachers of the deaf. This shows how much work was done to convince people that the resolution was something that was needed and that it was not going to break the bank. Of course, the bank was thought to be a little bigger than it turned out to be.

Let me quote you the resolution. It is a little long, but I believe it is so important in the work being done that it perhaps should be on the wall in offices where these problems are dealt with so that all can read it.

WHEREAS, there are individuals with hidden disabilities, and WHEREAS, the needs of these individuals with hidden disabilities have not been addressed at Workshop IV; THEREFORE BE IT RESOLVED THAT the Social Concern Workshop IV recommends that the "discrete handicapped" be included in mainstreaming as far as providing services and facilities necessary to permit said handicapped persons to live their lives to the fullest potential possible.

WHEREAS, the White House Conference on Handicapped Individuals is designed to consider the needs of all United States citizens affected by handicapping conditions, and

WHEREAS, The conference is described as addressing "the aspirations, abilities, and problems of physically and mentally disabled Americans of all ages. . .," and

WHEREAS, the classifications "physically" and "mentally" have created some uncertainty and confusion among the conference delegates, particularly as those terms relate to neurological impairments such as epilepsy, autism, and certain communicative disorders, and

WHEREAS, under the general classifications of "physically and mentally disabled," other hidden handicaps such as cystic fibrosis, diabetes, neoplastic diseases and other handicapping medical disorders are included as physical disabilities, and

WHEREAS, this fact requires clarification and emphasis since public opinion generally perceives of physically handicapped individuals as persons who have orthopedic impairments or other obvious handicapping conditions;

NOW, THEREFORE BE IT RESOLVED that the White House Conference on Handicapped Individuals reaffirms and

emphasizes that neurological impairments and other handicapping medical disorders are considered to be physical
handicaps under the classifications used at the White House
Conference on Handicapped Individuals, and

BE IT FURTHER RESOLVED that the White House Conference on Handicapped Individuals is of the opinion that the
discernible or "hidden handicaps" should receive equitable
consideration throughout the deliberations of this Conference by all workshops, caucuses, delegations, and sessions,
and that the final report reflect their deliberations to ensure
that the needs of persons disabled by these conditions are
not overlooked in resultant planning and services for the
handicapped in the United States of America, and

BE IT FINALLY RESOLVED that the substance of this
resolution be included in the final report of this Conference
to be submitted to the President and the United States Congress, and also in the implementation plan of the White
House Conference.

Properly understood, this is a radical resolution. Before, the
outcome of a disease *led* to the handicap. Here the concept is
introduced that the disease itself *is* the handicap. Look at the
secretary with Hodgkin's disease. She looked the same as you or I
when I spoke to her. She had no problem with her stamina during
the day, but the disease itself was the handicap for her. Many
times the treatment of the disease is the handicap. Chemotherapy
for cancer not only affects the cancer, but affects the whole body.
In my capacity as consultant for the Texas Rehabilitation Commission I am often confronted with claims based upon the fact
that persons are receiving therapy that they find debilitating and
accordingly they cannot work. This I think is a valid claim. It is
not a permanent handicap, but certainly a temporary handicap.

Let me change pace here and add a word of warning about all
this. I think the hidden handicap and the resolution's recognition
of it as a legitimate condition deserving of special programs,

consideration by rehabilitation commissions, presents both an opportunity and a danger. I was very concerned that the Secretary recognized alcoholism as a disabling condition. I know that since the Easter decision, alcoholism is recognized for criminal purposes as a disease. And yet, in our minds, and in most people's minds, the feeling is that "on our own volition" is a casual factor in such condition. There is some element of a personal contribution to alcoholism, personal responsibility. If one can still use such a phrase, alcoholism is seen by most people as being part medical problem and part bad habit. It is different from the hidden handicaps envisioned by the resolution because here the disease process is completely beyond the control of the affected person. Alcoholism may be a disease, but it is obviously a different form of disease from typhoid fever and lupus.

The disease processes discussed in the resolution, such as epilepsy, diabetes, cystic fibrosis, and neoplastic diseases, are afflictions for which the patient has no role in the pathogenesis. Schizophrenia and other functional psychoses are clearly physical in origin and are obviously distinguishable from personality problems such as neuroses. It must be the goal of those working with patients with hidden handicaps to make sure the public, legislators, and other decision makers realize that these are ultimately grounded in physical illness and that though the disabling aspect may be perceived as subjective, it is grounded in an objective reality, a discernible disease process.

I wish I could end this discussion with a glowing summary of all the advances that have been scored since the passage of the resolution on hidden handicaps by the White House Conference. As you know, things have changed a lot in the last few years. Perhaps we are in a phase where we must digest many new concepts that have only recently been accepted. Maybe the White House Conference represented a high point and now we are in an epoch of diminished expectations. Only time will tell where we go from here. But this does not diminish the importance of the resolution. A large number of delegates, most all of whom were chosen by handicapped individuals and who were almost handicapped or relatives of the handicapped, strongly endorsed this resolution.

There is always value in telling the truth even though nothing perceptible or measurable comes from it. The resolution is on the books for all to see, and in time it will have an impact. As its existence becomes more widely known and its acceptance more general, we will see changes. For the time being, if it only gives recognition to those with hidden handicaps and lets them know of society's awareness of the paradoxical problem, it has served a valuable purpose and the work that went into it has been worthwhile.

REFERENCES

1.   Webster's Third New International Dictionary of the English Language. Springfield, Mass.: G. & C. Merriam Company, 1968.
2.   Bartholome, W. G. Good intentions become imperfect in an imperfect world. Proceedings of the Fifth Annual Mental Health Conference, Reintegration of the Medically Exceptional Child, Houston, Texas, April 25-26, 1980. These proceedings, pp. 17-33.

CHAPTER 12

The Problem as Experienced by Teachers

ALLISON STOVALL

This discussion focused on the problem of reintegrating the medically exceptional child from the standpoint of the teacher. Clearly the teacher confronted with mainstreaming these children has sensed the awesome nature of the task before her. When teachers are asked to meet the needs of special children without being given adequate preparation, they are often anxious. This is particularly so for the teacher who meets with 150 students each day. Discipline problems in large classes often prevent the teacher from being able to give enough individual attention to children with medical problems.

The teacher's confidence in her ability to work with these children is crucial to success. A teacher can be more comfortable when she has information about the child's needs and abilities. Teachers need the collaboration of parents, nurses, and students to be effective. Parents need to serve as liaisons between the health care providers and the schools. They can interpret their children's needs and abilities with authority. For example, parents' visits to teachers prior to the start of classes in the fall can allay anxieties of all parties and provide a happier school experience for the student. Problems arise in those cases where parents do not contact the school due to indifference or embarrassment.

The teacher looks to counselors, nurses, and home school community agents to aid her in working with children and their parents. School nurses are critical as interpreters of medical data to counselors and teachers. Counselors aid in placing children with the appropriate class groups and in disbursing pertinent data on their needs to school personnel. The schools rely on home school community agents to contact families in the community who are reluctant to contact the school.

Creative teachers find ways to include students in attending to the needs of special children. After the exceptional child has been adequately informed regarding his medical status, he can help the other students to understand. At times, an articulate student can put his classmates at ease by explaining his cancer or his seizure disorder to them with the teacher's support. Thereafter, he garners support from his peers.

The school environment plays an important part in the adaptation of the medically exceptional child. Two parents in our group had particularly positive experiences when the school community rallied to support them when it was learned their daughter had brain cancer. When she moved from that small elementary school to a junior high school of 2,000 students, she did not receive the attention that her parents wanted for her. Upon hearing of the extension of the middle school concept from the school administrators among us, they were disturbed to learn of sixth-grade children having seven different teachers a day. While the social and academic developmental issues may be met more appropriately in a middle school program of transition, the size of the school makes it more difficult for the special child to get the necessary attention.

Part of the problem for the patient-student and family is fading: the lesson in reality that awaits them in school and in the community. Educators, parents, and health care personnel have high ideals for the care of children. At times, our children encounter unkindness, indifference, fear, and hostility from peers or personnel in school. While this creates discomfort for the child and family, it must be recognized that children need to deal with these realities.

Although the school system may have numerous programs to address the needs of these special children, the efficacy of the programs is questionable if they are not tailored to individual needs. If a home-bound program cannot include the child who is chronically ill but is absent from school for less than the required four weeks when under treatment, then that program needs to be revised. If ARD conferences are held less often than recommended, parents have difficulty communicating their concerns regarding their children's progress in school. Flexibility is required if the partnership among hospital, patient, family, and school is to lead to optimum reintegration of medically exceptional children.

CHAPTER 13

Why Teachers?
The Reminiscences of a
Discussion Leader as Parent

CHARLES R. SHAW

For me, this conference had a special significance, a special importance I hadn't anticipated. Looking over the program in advance, I hadn't appreciated that the conference was a collaboration between us medical people and educational people. But there they were, teachers, principals, school counselors, superintendents. It was a fine idea, getting us together, those of us who care for the medical problems of children and those who care for children and help them to grow up well. We have much in common, much to communicate about, much to help each other with.

I was lucky to have had a good initial experience with my first grade teacher, a sweet lady, who cared about children and was sensitive to our feelings. I remember how much I wanted to please her. It wasn't one of those childhood crushes; I don't even remember what she looked like. But I remember she made me want to please her, made me feel good when I was able to please her. And I learned quickly that the best thing to do was to learn the lessons well, spell the words correctly, do things right academically; it was a great way to start off in the academic world.

I didn't realize at the time, of course, what effect she was having. Perhaps the first time I came to appreciate that was in reading James Hilton's novel, *Goodbye Mr. Chips,* when I was in high school. His new young wife, Cathy, was talking about how

pleased she was that Chips was a teacher: "Oh, Chips, I'm glad you
are what you are. I was afraid you were a solicitor or a stock-
broker or a dentist or a man with a big cotton business in Man-
chester. When I first met you, I mean. Schoolmastering is so
different, so important, don't you think? To be influencing those
who are going to grow up and matter to the world." Chips said he
hadn't thought about it like that, at least not often. He did his
best; that was all anyone could do in his job. "Yes, of course,
Chips. I do love you for saying simple things like that."

Later, when my own daughter was in school, I would go to the
parent-teacher meetings, talk with the teachers, and feel a sense of
humility and gratitude. They were so important to her, so important in helping her grow up well. Most of them, then, were
younger than I, and looked up to me as a doctor, as the father of
a pupil. I used to smile inwardly sometimes, amused that they
were not aware of my sense of humility, almost worshipfulness.
And later, working as a child psychiatrist, consulting with the
teachers and principals, trying to work out among us how to deal
with this or that troubled child. I again had a great sense of
respect for the teachers, the ones who were dealing every day,
every hour with these problems, with these difficult children,
with parents who were sometimes less than helpful, less than
understanding.

The title of this chapter is not original with me; it was cribbed
from a chapter Marie Rasey wrote, a great educator whom I was
privileged to know shortly before she died. The point she was
making, in a book on *The Nature of Man,* was that a function of
teachers is to provide an ego ideal, that this is usually more important than their academic teaching, that it is the main reason
why teachers must be mature and insightful persons and why they
can never be replaced by audiovisual aids.

Well, it's still true, of course, more true than ever, in fact, as
times become more complex and parents seem to have less time
for their children. So often, the day a child enters school is the
first day he has the experience of being treated as a person by an

adult. It is an enormous responsibility, this influence these teachers bear.

And now, with the new law, Public Law 94-142, teachers have even more responsibility. As if the load were not enough, dealing with the reasonably intact and competent children, they now are saddled with the additional load of handicapped children, all kinds of handicapped children: deaf, retarded, paralyzed, dying of cancer, living with cancer. Being naive, being out of touch with recent developments in this burgeoning field, I had no idea what had been going on, what was developing. It took me awhile, most of the first day of the meeting, to comprehend the dimensions of this revolution. And, through most of the sessions, while functioning as a discussion leader, I was mainly a discussion listener. I was learning, learning a great deal.

What did I learn? Well, among other things, that they are coping. As always, most of them are coping. They have this responsibility, this concern, and they take on the load. Just a little more. It's the way they operate, always have. Not without complaining, not without some resentment. They are, for the most part, not altruists or martyrs, but responsible people. They are very concerned, sometimes angry, that the budget is going to be cut back. Some of the counselor staff may be reduced, and just when they are needing more. But most of them refuse to consider that the new law is a bad law. I tried to bring this out. I even took the side that it is a bad law, for awhile. I even believed that, for awhile; in fact, I am still not altogether convinced which way it should be. It took a lot or reorientation in my own thinking, processing that is still going on, that it's better for the handicapped, the retarded, to be in school with the "normal." It just doesn't apply to the old traditional thinking. And thinking changes slowly.

When I was a child psychiatrist in Michigan years ago, I saw many problem children, the learning disabled, the handicapped. I used to deal with them, working with the school people, getting them into special classrooms with special education teachers. Some of them, the more severe, would be admitted to the inpatient unit, the children's psychiatric hospital where they were taught in small groups, small classrooms, all under special education teachers. Some of them, the ones that did well, were gradually rehabilitated back to public school. But it was a slow, difficult process. Now, here, the idea is that all of the children, the handicapped of all kinds, should be integrated into a regular classroom. I still don't know. I would need to see more of the results to be convinced. But the idea that the regular school system has responsibility for these kids, that I can accept.

The lines had been drawn the very first morning of the conference, the two introductory talks, polarized, the one by a doctor, pessimistic, cynical, deliberately inflammatory, that "we can't force the world to be a therapeutic community," that about the best we can expect is to train these handicapped to "pass" for normal. Then the lawyer, the optimist, a bit idealistic, who talks to the educators, perhaps never sees the classrooms or the children, is convinced that the law is good, that compulsory education laws constitute "the very foundation of our free society," is convinced that the system is working well, that it's right, fair, good, that all handicapped should have equal opportunity.

In one of the sessions, we talked about equal opportunity, considered that it's not the same thing as the full realization of every person's innate capacities. There is a basic conflict. Realization of one's capacities can sometimes cost an inordinate amount of money, and of time spent with teachers, with special programs; others, with high capacity, innate capability, can run almost without teachers, almost without costing the state anything. What is right? What is fair? Is it fair to take the money from teaching normal children and spend most of it on raising the handicapped to a slightly higher level of capability? Some of the teachers showed that they hadn't really thought about the issue in these terms. Some didn't want to think about it.

We talked about the responsibility of teachers to the children and to society. Trying to get perspective, we went back to the beginning of compulsory education laws in this country. I read an excerpt from a textbook I authored on child psychiatry.

> In the days when Tom Sawyer went to the old one room schoolhouse in Missouri, a guiding principle of education was spare the rod and spoil the child. If Mark Twain's accounts are to be credited (he *has* been suspected of exaggeration), children went to school grudgingly, hated it heartily, and envied Huckleberry Finn, son of the town drunk, who remained free. In those days, children who were tempermentally or intellectually unsuited to attend school, or who were needed to support the family, simply stayed at home. Today, if a child does not go to school, the parents can be legally prosecuted.
>
> There are a number of landmarks in the history of child psychiatry, but perhaps the most significant was the passage of compulsory education laws. The requirement that all children attend school had a number of sweeping effects. One was to demonstrate and at times to aggravate the multitude of mental and emotional problems among the juvenile population. Another was to force attention and effort to care and treatment of these problems.

The new public law is thus seen as a logical continuation of the compulsory education laws. There will be tensions and dislocations. It will put severe loads and pressures on the school system, on some of the children, the normal as well as the handicapped. There will be times and situations when the wisdom of the law will be doubted. But the consensus, as drawn from this meeting, from people who are in the midst of the system and who are watching it operate, is that it will grow and will succeed.

We who deal with medically ill children, particularly children with cancer, have some of our own doubts as well as some of our own optimism. It was encouraging, at this meeting, to see how well along the educators are coming in their understanding, and I find myself wanting to understand better how to help these misfortunate children in getting along, in being assimilated into the society of normal children. We know from talking with our patients that they want most of all to be treated as normal; they do not want to be considered apart, freaks, persons to be avoided. It is exciting to be a part of this scene. This is clearly a new era in child oncology. So many of the children are staying around, are continuing to live and to function. It was, in some ways, much simpler when they simply went ahead and died and we could mourn them for a while and go on our ways. Now they are staying, partly because of our own endeavors. We have the responsibility, we and their teachers.

Section IV

THE SOLUTION

Introduction

VIRGINIA THOMPSON

At this conference, we have been examining the needs of the medically exceptional child. We have heard special educators say, "We need more special programs." Wait, our focus slipped a little there.

We have heard a lawyer say, "The law requires. . . ." Does that blur our image further?

We have heard patients say, "We need special services." The child seems to be slipping away.

Have we really focused on the needs of the child? What services do we offer and who is the consumer? Who decides what the consumer needs? To bring things into perspective, we have Elizabeth Deuble, Principal of Sinclair Elementary School.

Mrs. Deuble has taught several grade levels and has served as coordinator of the Houston Independent School District's Career Education. She organized and implemented one of the district's magnet schools. For the past several years she has been the principal of an elementary school with a large population of handicapped children and she has worked with a special team of educators whom she calls "talented and dedicated people who care about children."

Can we make that which is imperfect perfect or can we adjust reality. Perhaps the solution is to adjust the patient and his environment to reality. To discuss this is Dr. Jan van Eys, Head of the Department of Pediatrics, The University of Texas System Cancer Center M. D. Anderson Hospital and Tumor Institute.

Dr. van Eys is a native of the Netherlands who arrived in Houston by way of Vanderbilt University and University of

Washington School of Medicine. In addition to oncology, as a pediatrician, Dr. van Eys is interested in nutrition, genetics, hematology, and mental health. He is a prolific writer and superb organizer of workshops, as evidenced by this, the Fifth Annual Mental Health Conference.

CHAPTER 14

The Child is the Consumer

ELIZABETH DEUBLE

It has been noted that for every complex problem there is a simple solution. And that solution is probably wrong. Historically, this has been in dealing with the "exceptional" child. Society for years chose to separate and alienate those who were different—out of sight, out of mind.

Society has now developed a collective conscience and has determined that these children, born across the strata of the populace, should be educated in the same environment as the normal child.

Consequently, reintegrating the medically exceptional child into the public schools is being done today with much flag-waving. We rattle off public law numbers and all sorts of acronyms such as ARD and IEP. We flinch at the mention of parent-advocacy groups. The interminable paperwork in the name of accountability and the ever changing interpretations and guidelines nearly require that a brace of Philadelphia lawyers be on retainer for anyone responsible for implementing the process.

We become system oriented. We develop "a way" to do things. We parade our army of good intentions through countless procedures, protecting our flanks at all times against "being out of compliance."

Now the child is at the schoolhouse door. We've been expecting him. The innumerable reports from physicians, psychologists, therapists, as well as from educators who have provided any academic interventions, have been read. We've had conferences with parents, as to their concerns and expectations. Yet, in all likelihood, this is our first meeting with the child. I have had this experience all too frequently.

We have the IEP (Individualized Educational Plan) prepared. We have fulfilled our legal and social obligations. But we don't know the child—a flesh and blood, living, breathing person with needs, feelings, and wants peculiar only to him. We have been in the habit of designing programs to be geared to some vague and nebulous "norms," rather than providing for these individual needs.

Targeting the individual needs relevant to the educative process for the medically exceptional child requires that the goal should be, in every instance, a total effort to guide and facilitate learning.

Learning environments play a significant role in meeting these needs. The physical environment has been recognized as an area of concern. Many schools have changed from massive foreboding institutions to informal and friendly structures in which the learner rather than the system is the central concern. Certainly we can have the appropriate specialized equipment adapted to the physical needs of the handicapped children, but that is not the environment. Equipment, in and by itself, is clinical and can create a hostile or sterile atmosphere.

I would like to cite an example. We have a teacher who has a colorful cardboard fireplace in a corner of her classroom. It is the kind you find in stores at Christmas with a Santa standing in front. When it is time for floor games or story telling, everyone gathers on the rug in front of the fireplace. Our wheelchair student can crawl on the rug and lounge with all the other children. It offers a warm, cozy, friendly atmosphere.

The intangible aspect of the intellectual-emotional environment exerts considerable influence. Attitudes and values held by people come into play. It is important to recognize that some people have a built-in apprehension and distaste for deviations from the norm.

The medically exceptional child can come in a wide assortment of variances from the norm. These are the children who are categorized as mentally retarded, speech impaired, learning disabled, physically handicapped, visually impaired, and emotionally or behaviorally disturbed.

These children must react to these attitudes and values. An inappropriate environment can effectively deter us from our desired goals and objectives.

Responsible leadership must anticipate this inevitable problem and be prepared to assist personnel to intercept the problem. In-service meetings and informal conferences with classroom teachers and support personnel prove beneficial. We try to press for the "I'm O.K., You're O.K." (1) syndrome. Use of the *TA for Kids* (2) (transactional analysis) philosophy is also effective.

While children are sometimes guilty of cruel taunting, it is usually abrogated through a matter-of-fact dissemination of accurate information about the problems and symptoms the handicapped child exhibits.

The establishment of these positive environments can only be accomplished through the interventions of the teacher. When we discuss the needs of the medically exceptional child, it is tantamount that we have exceptional teachers. Even in the most ideal circumstances, teaching is one of the most demanding professions that exists. Handicapped children profoundly need teachers who basically respect the individuality of children. They need teachers who are facilitators of learning rather than simply sources of knowledge. The concept of the teacher as the "fountain of knowledge" has outlived its day. If the adage is true that we live in an environment that is continually changing, it is even truer for those dealing with medically exceptional children. We are faced with an entirely new situation in education where the goal of education, if these children are to survive, is the facilitation of change and learning. The only child who will be educated is the child who has learned how to learn. It is the only basis for security for these youngsters.

In a system in which facilitation of learning is a primary goal, the classroom teacher will necessarily have to devote major attention to the "individual" learner. All educational decisions as they relate to expectations have to be made with the learner, or if you will, the consumer of the educative process, foremost in mind. Not to overlook the obvious, we must state that these teachers require a high degree of expertise in working with people. They take on an added dimension of a guidance role within such a framework. It becomes a matter of helping each student to become informed about his progress and problems and the next steps to be undertaken.

Learners are best motivated to pursue a goal when they perceive the goal as worth striving for and when they can receive gratification in the process. It is imperative that the teacher ensures that the attainment of the goal, by these youngsters in particular, is feasible.

Encouragement is one of the most vital needs of any corrective effort. A retreat from progress will find its beginnings in discouragement, particularly in childhood.

Parents and teachers alike must develop skills needed to encourage children. One of the problems involved in beginning a task is that of motivation or overcoming inertia. This task is difficult enough in its own right, but it is enormously worsened if the student is handicapped. He can be overwhelmed by the full scope of the task set before him. Oftentimes a child can be induced to eat when a small portion is put before him; just so, a student can more often be stimulated to work by a reasonable partial assignment than by the assignment of a whole task at once.

We cannot expect progress, however, unless we recognize that the child needs the assistance of encouragement. It is necessary to make him feel his worth and therefore feel secure.

Some aspects of the encouragement process are worth noting. First, make the child feel that she is the kind who can do it. It's all right to try. Failure is no crime. Second, provide plenty of opportunities for successful achievement. Don't set standards so high that the child is constantly falling short. Third, be pleased with a reasonably good attempt. Show confidence in her abilities.

Fourth, accept the child as she is. Like her as she is so she can like herself. It is important to remember that children have certain rights and privileges. I feel that one of these rights is recognition for effort. In effect, we must not let the tail wag the dog. While we most definitely are responsible for the proper implementation of Public Law 94-142, and while we werlcome parental involvement, that is not the bottom line. What we do with the child in the school setting is.

I have touched on a few needs such as the physical and the intellectual-emotional environment, the need for skilled, but more important, sensitive teachers, and use of the encouragement process. There are many other specific needs that could be mentioned, but I suspect they will fall into one of those categories.

I cannot leave this topic without a further comment about the parents. They are as diverse as the children. And we work with all of them. There are the parents who proclaim, "Aha, now we have a law; it is ours and we are going to squeeze every drop out of it, whether or not it really applies to our child." There are the concerned parents who are involved, supportive, and helpful. They are the ones who create a "team" situation with the school and with whom one can communicate in a give and take manner. There are parents who go through the motions. They will show up at an ARD (Admission Review and Dismissal) meeting. They will say, "I can't do a thing with him. Anything you want to try is O.K." They will sign their name to the signature page of the document and leave. There are also those parents who are impossible to contact, whose list of excuses for nonattendance reads like a list in *The Guinness Book of World Records,* and who could, frankly, care less. They are delighted for the school to handle the problem. Knowing the state of parental care and involvement becomes an integral part of our establishing the emotional environment for the child.

Permit me a personal example of one of the most meaningful parental relationships a principal can enjoy. When I became a principal in mid-September two and a half years ago, we enrolled a cerebral palsied child. She had just returned to the Houston Independent School District from the Cerebral Palsy Center. The parents were totally opposed to this. Their previous experience with public schools had been painful. They wanted Kelly kept in the protected environment of the Cerebral Palsy Center. The Center wisely said that this child could benefit more from a regular school setting, even if Kelly was self-contained in a generic classroom. The father was fighting mad and the mother was a bundle of nerves. I was naive. We went through stages, to be sure, but let me tell you where we are now. Our trust level for each other is impregnable. Sue, Kelly's mother, is going to be PTA president this next year. How about that for reintegration of the parent of the medically exceptional child!

Sue and I have held each other in both tearful and joyful embraces about Kelly and her ups and downs. Tom, a prominent businessman and a very protective father, has vowed both to me and to the General Superintendent of H.I.S.D. that he would be happy to testify in our behalf, in a court of law if necessary, as to the positive aspects of having Kelly in our school. Sue has been very busy of late with her PTA duties and working with all the other parents or at school functions. She is a fulfilled, vivacious lady, far different from the single-faceted person I first met. But who has benefited from all this? Kelly, of course! Her independence and self-confidence have grown beyond every stretch of our imagination. Two years ago she could not walk into a room with two strangers in it. The other night she faced an audience of a couple hundred strangers, and as her mother was installed as president, Kelly smiled and waved and charmed these people. It was her night. We must see past the forest to the trees, for children like Kelly are the young saplings to nurture.

We now must ask ourselves about the role the student plays in the scheme of things. I contend that their personal involvement in improving the teaching/learning process is a big step in the right direction. It is our commitment to encourage this process. Students must come to believe that their input is valued and expected, no excuses and no patronization. They cannot slough off because of their handicap. They must be participants, not spectators.

As we work toward helping these children become self-advocates, we must help them learn to discern the difference between becoming demanding, self-seeking individuals and becoming persons who have developed strategies that will help them grow to their fullest potential and to transfer skills learned in school to adult life.

I want to emphasize that the editorial "we" that I'm using refers to the efforts of the teachers. It is they who with the patience of Job make things happen.

Little happenings mean a lot when working with medically exceptional children. When you are trying to develop their self-confidence to the point where they can take over some of the direction of their lives as most normal children do, there are many pitfalls. For one thing, give students time to respond. Many of the handicapped children are not given the chance to intercede in their own behalf simply because we do not give them enough time to respond. It may take them longer to speak and to make themselves understood. Their articulation may be poor, their modulation may be weak, and they may struggle to verbalize. Be patient. Listen to them. Don't look at your watch. Don't shut them off with an "uh-huh" or a shrug.

Students can be effective change agents (3) and committees can be an effective way to make things happen. It was through the efforts of one of our handicapped youngsters, a class delegate, that the Health Council recently dropped its annual tasting luncheon where each child on the council participates in creating a lunch from the four basic food groups. Instead, she recommended and the Health Council adopted a resolution that they all assist in making the general lunch session more enjoyable. They made posters and went from class to class to lead discussion groups to get their points across. It all started with an idea from Janet. Working on committees will be successful when decisions are reached by consensus.

If children are to become self-advocates, it is up to us to help them to be comfortable with the unknown and willing to take risks. If they are to become intercessors for themselves, they must study new ways to solve problems. We must assist them in focusing on personal development to offset any handicap they might have. Youngsters need to develop their creative processes. They must recognize that learning is a lifelong process to meet varying changes and needs. In addition to learning how to learn, they must learn how to generate ideas. They must learn how to accommodate, adapt, and cope with changing situations and unforeseen circumstances. In many instances these children can utilize adaptive education to replace straight cognitive learning, and they can do so very effectively. It is a class example of a child acting as an intercessor in his own behalf. Profound thinkers are those who are sought out because of their healthy, productive personalities and not necessarily their able bodies. History will testify to that.

Remember that mainstreaming is a reality! Remember, too, that the basic principle underlying mainstreaming is that handicapped students can benefit educationally and socially from being in programs with nonhandicapped students. Mainstreaming is based on the assumption that handicapped children have more similarities than differences in comparison with their nonhandicapped peers.

When talking about management, it cannot be said that learning can take place only in *this* setting and not in *that* setting, or that learning can best be achieved only under *these* conditions and not under *those* conditions. Some learning can—and may—take place anywhere in almost any setting and within an almost limitless range of conditions.

Within the existing system of education, virtually all responsibility for high quality and productive learning experiences is placed upon the individual classroom teacher. Typically, the teacher is in charge of and almost totally responsible for all of the essential factors and procedures that facilitate learning.

Students, therefore, must rely upon the good fortune and/or management of the system if they are to have access to teachers who possess the attributes needed to develop procedures designed to bring about optimum learning.

I doubt that any teacher can meet all of the demands made upon her. Producing all of the desired learner outcomes from our young consumers at a reasonable level of efficiency is a near impossibility. The teacher must rely on the support services organized to assist in the management: nurses, counselors, diagnosticians, materials specialists.

I would like to list a few characteristics necessary to ensure effectiveness in placing emphasis upon the student. First, the student should be encouraged and helped to be in a position, and continuously in a frame of mind, to accept the responsibility for her own learning. Knowledge is something she herself must acquire, not that which is "shoved down her throat." Second, a student needs to be helped to accept the objectives of instruction as her own goals. Therefore, the objects are defined in terms that are understood by her. Third, performance measures should be designed primarily to permit the student to demonstrate her acquired competencies and not merely test her inadequacies. Fourth, the curriculum should be sequential to provide continuous progress, but individual alternatives within the instruction should be made available to each student.

Yes, we've had some success stories at Sinclair Elementary School—some more so than others. However, the final chapters have yet to be written on these youngsters. Not only are the results of the race not in yet, we are not even near the finish line. We will continue to provide the consumer with the supply he needs with the hope that our good intentions will become less imperfect in our sincere effort to do what is right.

REFERENCES

1. Harris, T. A. I'm OK—You're OK. New York: Harper & Row, 1969.
2. Freed, M., Freed, A. TA for Kids. Sacramento, Calif.: Malmar Press, 1977.
3. Wright, J. Students can be effective change agents. Educ. Dig., May 1979, pp. 48–50.

CHAPTER 15

Changing the World is Not the Best Solution

JAN VAN EYS

INTRODUCTION

Every child ought to feel unique. Every child is unique. The greatest success in child rearing occurs when parents succeed in instilling that reality. To feel unique is to feel self-assured, to be able to utilize unique potential without fear of negative comparison. Therefore, every child ought to feel exceptional. But that is not what occurs. There is enormous pressure to be only exceptional in flashes, but not in general. To be a genius is suspect, to be overtly exceptional is considered eccentric.

The use of the word "exceptional" has become even more burdened and thereby changed into a suspected label when it started to be used as a euphemism for handicap. Concepts have become so confused that being exceptional by being outstanding is even suspect.

To be exceptional means that the average, the usual, does not apply. When being exceptional is, in fact, a handicap, an indication of performance below the average, there are two options: The concept average can change or the individual can change. The first sounds at face value absurd, but that is what the exceptional individuals are beginning to expect. As the concept exceptional has changed, so has the concept average changed from a mathematical one into a label to be decried and abused. This paper will attempt to bring into focus the challenge for the exceptional individual in

129

an average society, and to bring the concept average back into perspective.

THE AVERAGE

Concepts will be illustrated largely from the obvious problems of the severely physically handicapped. Cancer as the hidden handicap is far more insidious, but fewer are familiar with its problems. It is an axiom to this reasoning that the problems are no different.

The Definition of Average

Average is a mathematical concept whereby one can define a population by the sum of the measurements of each individual divided by the number of individuals. If the group is evenly distributed, this describes the population partially. If one further describes the population by determining the extent of extremes, usually expressed by the statistical concept of standard deviation, one has a good measure of the population. Only when the measurements are extremely unequally distributed over the population, that is, when the distribution is skewed, the average is not the same as the median, which is the measurement that divides the population into two equal groups. However, when we talk about societies containing large numbers of individuals, such distinctions fade. Almost no measure of large groups of individuals is so skewed that the average and median diverge. When you talk about an exceptional child, the whole United States population of the same age is the peer group against which exceptionality is defined. It is quite possible to limit the comparison to smaller and smaller subsets until no exceptionality remains. However, that is counterproductive because that accentuates the exceptionality by grouping it. The ambition of every physically handicapped child is to become a counselor of the similarly handicapped. By making that the uniform focus of such children, we would, in fact, group them outside society. As a first approximation we need to compare the handicapped against society as a whole. However, there are many types of measurements that can be applied to a population to use as a yardstick by which a child could be measured as exceptional. These could be grouped as concrete averages, accomplishment averages, and averages of being.

Concrete Averages

To avoid societal chaos there must be a physical description of the population. For instance, knowing the average size and spread of people makes the clothing industry profitable. It simply would not be feasible to have the waste of providing all sizes in equal quantity, regardless of necessary or even sybaritic consumption. To be exceptionally tall or short, or to be exceptionally shaped, imposes a real and significant burden. But the cost of any item of clothing would be prohibitive if each store were to stock all eventualities. That is why we have shops entitled "Abundantly Yours" for the upper extremes in weight distribution. The average is not a label, but a description. In the same way we need the average size to design airplanes. We need the average intelligence to make the world function. If we did not know the average intelligence, traffic signs might be too difficult. If that were the case, traffic accidents would be orders of magnitude more frequently. We need to know the average age of the population to plan the number of schools, and thereby the totality of resources needed. We need to know the extremes to make a decision on the extremes of services. Such data collection is neither good nor bad. It is neither destructive nor constructive. That is the way the world is and that is the way the world needs to be described. To call the night black is no racial slur, but a statement of color.

To be exceptional means that one has to conquer the world described by such averages. The averages exist and they are what they are, not only because of the normals. Each exceptional child contributes equally to the average, with a one child/one unit equality. Removing the exceptional child from the total used to calculate the average would describe a world that is not real unless the exceptional child is ignored and cast out. In spite of the threat of ever more isolation, it is becoming customary to identify some subset that allows children, who are overall outside the limit of two standard deviations of the average, to be more like an identified set of peers. It follows that there will emerge a population subset that is largely below average. It also follows that the norms set by the remainder in the original population are now higher. The result is that improvement goals are harder to attain. If we then label the new subset with a term like "minorities," we have accomplished the ultimate segregation. The fact that almost 80 percent of Houston Independent School District children are members of minorities does not strike anyone as a strange perversion of language. It means, however, that we have suddenly generated a whole mechanism of finding reasons why a child is below average. If that were descriptive, that would be very good. But it usually is not just descriptive; it is trying to explain and thereby excuse. To be a member of a minority means that meeting the standards of that subset can be expected. The society is then told to accept the whole group because of their minority status. Then it is considered acceptable for the children to keep their low standard. I submit to do that is manipulation of children.

Accomplishment Averages

To set standards for societal performance that are the norm for a group is to accept the whole group as is. We generate societal expectations for a subset that are only commensurate with their own expectations. There is undoubtedly innate ability in children.

To argue otherwise is simply nonsense. There are, however, also varying degrees to which potential is realized. Very few children are overachievers. By setting the average of a particular subset, in which the exceptional child is comfortable, as the norm, and thereby as an excuse for a substandard level of performance, the child simply will never realize his potential.

The average norms for population as a whole are real. They are, by definition, as often exceeded as unmet. But society as a whole is determined by the average, until and unless one accepts fragmentation. There is, of course, a concept of unacceptable exceptionality. In other words, the members comprising the average determine a society that can tolerate certain exceptions only as overt exceptions. The obvious example of that situation is language. A single language is the norm of a society, even if the presence of multiple mother tongues is recognized. However, the moment a country is made officially bilingual it has begun to fragment. Countries like Canada and Belgium are at significant risk of disintegration. Even Switzerland can remain united only by allowing the largest possible autonomy to single language Kantons, and still, German is strongly dominant over French, Italian, and Roman. To allow a subset to speak only their own, nondominant language generates a suppressed minority. Teaching in early grades in such a language to communicate certain concepts does not solve the problem because the quality of later performance through a common language is totally dominant over those determined by average learning accomplishments. To be separated in a subculture precludes many of otherwise achievable accomplishments.

There is an accomplishment average. Knowledge is necessary, communication is necessary. To reject such average as unrealistic for certain exceptional children is rejecting such children from society. The vague hope that thereby society will change is unrealistic. Society either disintegrates or encompasses everyone. A small minority simply becomes rejected if it does not participate in setting the average. There is no limit to how much exceptionality is acceptable as long as the average norm is acceptable to the exceptional individual.

Averages of Being

In all these objective norms of average there is still a diversity of individuals. The participation towards establishing the norm is determined by an average of being. The feeling of being able to participate in society is the first necessity for all of us—whether we are exceptional or not. Society does not tolerate ill health, in body or in spirit. Society does not owe anyone, because one truly participates in society only when one is not in need of individual attention. A herd protects each member, but a sick member is rejected. A sick member in the herd simply cannot be protected because the mode of protection is normalcy. That may be swiftness for antelopes, ferocious behavior for baboons, or random exposure through quantity in schools of fish, thereby minimizing the risk of any one individual.

Humans do not need such physical protection anymore. But humans still need normalcy to survive in society. The average behavior of all societies with quantitatively insignificant exceptions is that of independent interdependent survival. No one is totally self-sufficient for all needs, but everyone is, after attaining a certain age, totally alone in adapting to society's behavior. If one does not earn a living, if one does not generate the wherewithal for good clothing and shelter, one can only survive by being a pariah. The ability to participate in society is purely dependent on one's self-image, within certain extreme limits.

There are, indeed, a few so mentally or physically limited or so mentally gifted that ordinary participation in society is not possible. The restrictions on the gifted do not concern us here, though such are as surely outside society as the mentally dull. Society must, however, set a lower limit of simplification for the handicapped and the bewildered beyond which it simply cannot go without endangering the total fabric. Such exceptionals are outside society. By their total dependency they do not contribute to the concept average, and they are accentuated in their exceptionality. There is a certain tyranny of the average that makes one react and demand that such rigid exclusion of exceptionality not be abused. However, no matter how one wants to avoid the problem, a limit does exist and must exist. Any accommodation at the lower end of the distribution curve will also accentuate the exceptionality of those at the other extreme.

For those who are exceptional within acceptable limits, the definition of acceptibility is largely one of mental health. There also is, in fact, an average of mental health, an average of being. That is the most divergent among societies. In a country like America, it is the most diverse in contribution towards the average. Nevertheless, there are norms that are expected before one can participate in society. Any serious deviation from such norms can be labeled mentally ill. It does not matter that such deviation is generated by real or even imposed physical exceptionality. One simply cannot communicate if the thought process is too foreign. Countries have gone to war because of misunderstandings of concepts. For better or worse, in our society it is the concept of self-sufficiency of nondependence that is incorporated in the concept of mental health. It is not an absolute but a dominant part of the self-concept. Good self-image and self-concept, a good view of potential, are the major components towards such mental self-sufficiency. It is simply inappropriate to approach a random fellow human with an outpouring of all the soul-troubling thoughts we may have. "How are you?" is not to be answered in exhaustive detail. In fact, mental health means one can answer truthfully "OK" to all except the most intimate. It simply means that one's personal problems do not interfere with one's ability to relate to fellow members in society.

Who Will Decide Unacceptable Exceptionality

There is then a limit of unacceptable exceptionality. When such limit is set, it is very variable from society to society and, in fact, from region to region. What is not acceptable in a harsh climate may be perfectly tolerable in another. Debilitating asthma generates total dependence, but a change in environment may totally negate this societal ostracizing.

The limits are set by both sides, society and the exceptional child. Society can indeed exercise a tyranny of handicap by imposing specific impossibilities on the exceptional. It is always possible to broaden the concrete average. To systematically block wheelchairs from access to the places where society gathers is declaring a limit that is totally arbitrary and imposed by a misplaced concept of the proper. It is no different from the despicable segregated restrooms of two decades ago. But it is reasonable to print newspapers with a vocabulary of the sixth grade and then to use the newspaper as a vehicle to disseminate instructions on how to participate in society. Anything simpler would so handicap the subtlety of meaning that it would result in a society that is a grey monotone of drabness.

However, as often as not, the limits are also set by the exceptional person. It is a major challenge to be exceptional and to know it. It is an even greater challenge to be exceptional and not realize it, except when one can rejoice in it. Anything short of that goal is a partial incorporation into society. That goal is rarely achievable, but it is a goal for all. Unfortunately, the fact that the average exercise a tyranny is often ignored because the average persons are afraid to expose their individual exceptionality.

THE EXCEPTIONAL CHILD

On the one hand, there is the great multitude composing society, and on the other hand, there is that one child who must become absorbed into that total, despite being patently different by some or other measure. It is a formidable task to carve out a lifestyle. Yet there is so much in the concept handicap that is relative that it ought not to be the formidable task that it is, provided a measure of mental health and independence is present or possible.

Physical Exceptionality

The relativity of exceptionality is most overt in the physical realm, which is also the most overtly abused area. This is because most of the physically average imagine that an unsound body is a sign of an unsound mind. In the past when life was simpler in concepts, malformed babies were simply rejected and abandoned. Later the "Dritter Reich," Hitler's Germany, rejected the Jews and gypsies as being unfit. While the concept was touted as a contamination of a super race by a group that was mentally inferior, the ultimate test to see if one was Jewish and thereby mentally unfit was the presence of circumcision.

But to be physically extreme is relative. The "little people," adults who have a genetic disease that results in extremely short stature, consider it an unacceptable genetic risk of a union between them has a significant probability of producing what most would call normal children. A normally sized child simply does not fit in a family of dwarfs. It is well to remember that even the most malformed child is composed of a number of cells that are so complex as to be biochemically near identical to those found in the average person. Physical exceptionality simply is relative.

Exceptionality and the Concept Handicapped

To be exceptional is a fact defined by the norm of society. It is a fact if one wants to be considered a member of a society. To be genetically male is a fact, to be six feet tall is a fact, to be a slow learner or to be a genius is a fact. All such realities can define the child as exceptional. But to have such exceptionality as a handicap is relative. Society and environment allow that since society is a homogeneity of diversity there is room for almost all. One simply has to select the niche that allows the exceptionality not to become a handicap. To be very tall becomes an asset as a professional basketball player and to be very short and light is an asset as a jockey. To be handicapped physically is often societally inflicted because of the concrete averages. But the average of accomplishment and the average of being are attainable by almost all simply because they are purely self-determined. Mental health cannot be achieved by changing all of society because that simply is not possible. Any attempt to achieve it is generating a certain handicap by the exceptional for themselves. Ultimately, when exceptionality becomes a handicap, it is the handicap of poor self-concept: the handicap of not asserting the rights of all individuals. It is true that the exceptional has to work harder to achieve that goal. That may not be considered fair, but to the question: "Why me?" there is only one retort: "Why not?" What has any one of us done to deserve a different fate than we received? Mythology abounds with stories of the undesirability of positive exceptionality. The poor who find that riches are as much a curse as a blessing, the subjects who find that responsibility is far more taxing than being led, the weak who find the expectations of the strong beyond endurance. Since time immemorial such lessons are taught and since time immemorial such lessons have failed to convince the exceptional. But to be a genius, to be disbelieved by all contemporaries, is more lonely than most physically exceptional can imagine. To have an exceptional memory can be a curse when all the convenient misremembering confronts you. To understand partially is a curse when the belief of all isolates you; yet the glimpse of the all fills the genius with the hopelessness of the unattainable. The striving for the unattainable is, in fact, accentuating the handicap of superior exceptionality.

Societal Guilt

Even when society allows the exceptional to participate, there is a vague concept of guilt about the fact that the exceptional child exists at all. Guilt is the poorest of drives to avoid the handicapping of the exceptional. Guilt does not allow equalization. It accentuates the exceptional by giving it a cause. To atone for the behavior of my ancestors towards other societal groups can be made an absurdity. It does not allow equal treatment, it only restores the absolute separation that existed in the past. Even the fostering of cultural imagery in minorities is only transiently helpful in generating a good image and is as much imposed by societal guilt over what was lost as it is positive. But societal guilt is so potent that it is fostered by the exceptional. They so often prey on this guilt to get what maybe their forefathers deserved but no longer now deserve. There is nothing more destructive to a child than undeserved praise and nothing generates undeserved praise more than guilt.

THE HANDICAP OF SELF-CONCEPT

Mental health is self-acceptance. That can be put as crassly as Huxley did in *Brave New World*, "Liking what you've got to do" (1), or it can be put as gently as a Sermon on the Mount. But it requires self-acceptance; acceptance of society does not suffice.

One of the most handicapped, yet still functional, young men I ever knew, wrote a book about his experiences (2). He was severely debilitated by cerebral palsy, yet he wrote:

Although educators, parents and the general public offer all the opportunities in the world for the handicapped, they *cannot* do everything for the individual nor can they make the person want to do for himself. Somehow there has to be motivation within the person. This motivation may not appear at the beginning. Discipline from educators and parents and self-discipline play a vital role in determining their success in life. These things are not usually considered pleasant. They may seem very harsh and unnecessary at the time, but the handicapped individuals will find that the discipline and self-discipline during their adolescent years become a great asset in accomplishing tasks and clearing hurdles late in life.

But if you had read this without knowing the exceptionality of the author, and if you changed the word "handicapped" to "adolescent," would you not think that this was the usual adult's admonishment to the teenager? Does not every teenager feel *"Weltfremd"*? Do they not all feel uniquely exceptional and frighteningly insecure—handicapped by the uncertainty? Only when they accept themselves will they begin to become adults. If they cannot find themselves, they never join society. They drift to Mission Beach in San Diego or similar subcultures where their exceptionality is average, but there their handicap is magnified by a collective inability to join society. There are, in fact, physical and legal obstacles to overcome for every adolescent that are as real as the lack of a wheelchair ramp.

In other words, almost all exceptionality is one of degree and not quantized. The limits imposed to participation in society are those imposed by the need for *independent* participation. Much of the perception of the exceptional child by society, in turn, is a reflection of the self-perception of the exceptional. If one says often enough I cannot do that, people will begin to believe you. And if society feels guilty enough, you have to say it only once to be believed. The more exceptional, the easier society believes you are handicapped and, in fact, wants to believe you are handicapped.

However, self-acceptance also means you do not practice self-delusion. The very short cannot really play professional basketball, and the very tall cannot really be a jockey. To be part of society does not mean that society has to fully accommodate you. We all have special needs—real or self-imposed. But that does not mean all of us should accept that limitation. If one wants to eat kosher foods, that is reasonable and proper, but others can eat ham. Such differences are neutral in the functioning of society. You have to accept yourself as you are. You have to accomplish something important in life to be at ease with yourself. You must not set unattainable goals because then you will never become satisfied with yourself. Nor should you abandon all goals because then you become excessively self-critical. No one can live with permanent failure.

Het Dorp

The principle of maximally accomplishing that which is possible is best illustrated by an experiment in Holland, called simply *Het Dorp,* the village. *Het Dorp* is an incorporated township in the Netherlands with a mayor, an elected town council, and all the services needed for a town—postoffice, store, police and fire protection. However, all inhabitants are exceptional. They are physically handicapped in the usual parlance. It is their village. They run it. They hire nonhandicapped support personnel. They are not supervised by nurses, but rather tell the nurses what *they* need. To a point, the exception is the average, but it is not a closed community. The township has equal standing in the Netherlands to all others. The members work inside or outside the town in regular society. They pay taxes locally and to the state and federal government. When my wife and I visited the town we were invited in a home. The girl who lived there had become near total quadriplegic as a young adult. At first she had resented the specialness of the place, but later found that she could live in *Het Dorp* as a normal person within the limitations that her exceptionality posed. Her physical limitation required her physical environment. But she achieved, thereby, an average of accomplishment and of being. Society did not adapt to her, she adapted to society. There were unattainable goals that were missed, just as there were memories of what could have been. But there was also maximal achievement within the achievable limits.

Despair

This contrasts with another experience, observed by Cavert School in Nashville, Tennessee, an institution for the multiply handicapped. The teenagers wanted to hold a dance, to be like other high school students. It was an unattainable goal. The dance was held, but it was an evening full of despair—despair of not willing to be oneself, as much as despair of willing to be what one is not (3). Imagining reality is not true reality. That does not mean that escapism is bad, but to escape in a land where reality is imitated is not the releasing escape of the fully imaginary.

POTENTIAL AND COMPLETENESS

No one can be everything or do all. Completeness is not an objectively attainable concept. To be a complete person only means a participation in society with certain freedoms of choice and self expression.

Martin McGrath has listed nine manifest needs for the handicapped:

Achievement —to do one's best, to be successful, to accomplish something important.

Deference —to get suggestions from others, to follow instructions, to do what is expected, to praise others, to accept leadership from others and to conform to customs.

Autonomy —to be able to come and go as desired, to say what one thinks.

Dominance —to argue one's point of view, to be a leader, to persuade and influence others, to supervise and direct others.

Nurturance —to help others, to treat others with kindness and sympathy.

Abasement —to feel guilty, when something goes wrong, to accept blame.

Change —to do something new and different, to meet new people, to have novelty and change in daily routine, to participate in new fads and fashions.

Heterosexuality —to engage in social activities with the opposite sex, to be in love.

Aggression —to attack one's point of view, to tell others off. (2) (pp. 34–35)

One might have chosen different words for the concepts, but the concepts are real for all of us. They come from a man who is very much handicapped, to a degree that one cannot easily imagine that independence could be possible.

But all elements of need that Martin McGrath quoted are only achieved when they are self-generated. No one can teach these elements. One can only help the exceptional child with mastering these enormous tasks. To express aggression with equanimity is hard for all of us; how much harder must it be for the severely handicapped?

It is quite possible that in the education process towards integrating the exceptional child the following concept must pertain:

> For education purposes . . . the crippled and other health impaired multiple handicapped population is seen as those individuals who as a result of physiological or functional disabilities, cannot have their educational needs met without specialized mediation, remediation, or modification of curriculum. (4)

But it does not follow that *goals* of education must be changed. Just because one is exceptional, society cannot be changed to remove exceptionality. To make aggression a nonnecessary need of the handicapped would mean to coddle the handicapped, to remove all obstacles, to generate a happiness as found in Huxley's *Brave New World*. That kind of happiness is indeed possible. But if one defines happiness that way, one ought to remember the words of the controller in *Brave New World*:

> Actual happiness always looks pretty squalid in comparison with the overcompensations for misery. . . . Being contented has none of the glamour of a good fight against misfortune, none of the picturesqueness of a struggle with temptation, or a fatal overthrow by passion or doubt. (1) (p. 265)

Self-determination would be lost. To generate a sexless society for the handicapped or the genetically burdened is a societal decision that equates tyranny and excommunication.

Of course, society does have prejudices. The concepts of the majority about the minority can be very skewed indeed. There must be attitude changes. The widespread held concept of the imminent death of the child with cancer must be changed. But it will, because it is an indisputable fact. When people do not die who are supposed to, you cannot ignore them. There is no fine line, but rather a chasm between teaching the public reality and making the public ignore reality to ignore the exceptional. To be complete on human terms, to achieve Martin McGrath's goals, one must cater to the individual. One cannot ask society to make such goals unnecessary. When we do, the handicapped will live in the *"Brave New World,"* even while the average do not.

THE OBLIGATION OF SOCIETY

There is in this dialectic conceptualization an idea of societal obligation towards all members of society. Such an obligation exists, but only by mutual consent and not by definition. Only for those who are accepted as human, but not yet as persons, is there an assumed obligation by society (5). That is routinely true for children, but that obligation implies dependency. That implies that there is no freedom to come and go, to be autonomous, to change independently. Once grown into adulthood, the exceptional child must have become an independent member of society.

Society as Business

Society, as the Western Democracies perceive it, is a collective business. We tax ourselves and buy services. We divide common labor, we generate protection, we decide on a minimally acceptable environment. Through that we consider that we make potential possible. Such an environment should, therefore, be the least restrictive possible to allow development of unusual potential. But society also dictates by the common acceptance of average, the constructive channels of potential development. A dependent human partakes of that society. But independent adults contribute to that society lest they lose their independence. Even temporary illness, paid for by self-selected third party payers, removes much of the independence of the individual.

Schooling as Obligation of the Individual

While school is an obligation of society, partaking of the opportunities inherent in school is the obligation of the individual. It was rarely said better than in the wisdom of Sirach:

> My child from your youth up cultivate education,
> And you will keep on finding wisdom until you are grey.
> Approach her like a man who plows and sows
> And wait for her abundant crops.
> For in cultivating her you will toil but little
> And soon you will eat her produce.
> She seems very harsh, to the undisciplined,
> And a thoughtless man cannot abide her.
> She will rest on him like a great stone to test him,
> And he will not delay to throw her off.
> For wisdom is what her name implies
> And to most men she is invisible. (6) (p. 234)

Later it states:

> My child, if you wish, you can be educated,
> And if you devote yourself to it you can become shrewd.
> If you love to hear, you will receive,
> And if you listen you will be wise. (6) (p. 235)

Our current laws do not state that to learn is a right—only the opportunity to learn. But to communicate one has to be able to speak. To speak one has to have words, and to have words one has to have concepts. It does not come automatically. Schools cannot teach beyond the capabilities of the child. Society has no obligation to assume independence where none exists. If independence is impossible, our society has decreed that dependence is allowed. Care will be given. But it is the *"Brave New World."* If the capability of the exceptional is limited by wanting to be helped rather than to help self, nothing is accomplished and independence is as surely unachievable as it is for the mentally incapable.

THE ADAPTATION TO SOCIETY

It follows, therefore, that one buys into society to become independent. Like any transaction, one may bargain about the price, but there is no independence possible unless the individual contributes to society independently. Society does act democratically in the sense that the average is determined by all who participate. To stay out of society, to ask support without contribution only results in not letting one's contribution help determine the average. Not so long ago a nation was excited by a young president who said:

> And so, my fellow Americans, ask not what your country can do for you: ask what you can do for your country. (7).

A similar spirit must be instilled into the exceptional child. That same president said:

> Man holds in his mortal hands the power to abolish all forms of human poverty and all forms of human life. And yet the same revolutionary beliefs for which our forebears fought are still at issue around the globe—the belief that the rights of

man come not from the generosity of the state, but from the hand of God. (7)

Whether we would have expressed it in such religious terms or in more humanistic or theosophical terms is irrelevant. But you cannot have it both ways. Reliance on the impersonal group that constitutes the average destroys the rights of being and individual on the terms in which we usually perceive them.

Everyone has a potential; therefore it ought to be magnified. However, the exceptionality *is* –it is a fact, not something to be ignored. The child must be helped to assimilate that fact. One must help to change what can be changed, accept what must be accepted, and one must learn one's limitation. Removing the limitation by improving the concept of average magnifies the handicap. That does *not* mean the physical limitations. Those are conceptually neutral. They are all very real, but do not generate the conceptual problems that are usually placed upon them. They are ultimately only important to the degree that they are used to prove the point of an unscalable obstacle of exceptionality. Eventually such barriers will come down, as soon as enough exceptional persons want to participate in society. But that is fundamentally different from insisting that society be adapted so that the exceptional does not need to struggle. To be exceptional is hard. It generates a struggle, nothing comes easy. The average accomplishments are hard to achieve; they are very far away for the exceptional child. If an average performance is what society demands to function, it should not be abandoned. But to state again: a goal for the handicap to teach and counsel other handicapped children is a removal from society, a modification of the exceptionality.

THE HIDDEN HANDICAP

Principles are best illustrated by the obvious. The physically exceptional child brings all problems into focus. But as already mentioned, even for them it is a matter of degree. The world can be cruel to them, by giving freedom one time and taking it away another time. The technology of the world progresses so rapidly that it is a major task to remain part of the world. To achieve entry will have been a formidable task for the exceptional children and it will remain ever so for them. But to so many of the older people the same applies. The average age in society is well below thirty years. Youth, vigor, and change for the sake of accomplishment of an individual abound.

The problem is compounded by the hidden handicaps. A physical deformity signals the exceptionality. But the perceived handicap is the most insidious. Having cancer, being depressed, the "If you only knew" syndrome, destroys more than cerebral palsy does. "Make my life tolerable, but do not ask me to change" is the common request. Society perpetuates such attitudes by generating imaginary excuses for slightly deviant behavior. It is a common fallacy that to have had cancer excuses one from achieving. To be blind excuses arrogant behavior, to be a diabetic sets up subtle blackmail.

It is bad enough to insist that society cater to the exceptional when the demand is, in part, as obvious as a physical complication of participation. It is self-destructive for exceptional children when they insist that society not only adapt, but must guess what the adaptation ought to be. It is devastatingly destructive when society complies and indeed tries to guess, usually with clues of prejudice and myth.

The best teacher of the exceptional child makes the child do for herself. The child with cancer is still a normal child (8) who needs to be challenged with expectations of accomplishments. To have cancer, to be exceptional, is not a label but a fact that must be dealt with. It is not a purifying suffering imposed by an inscrutable God, but it is the way one is. Any attitude from our part to foster another attitude is setting the child up for destruction and excommunication from society.

CONCLUDING REMARKS

It follows then that we must teach children to accept themselves and to be themselves. It is irrelevant that it is difficult, that most adults are not always capable of doing it. That does not make it any more reasonable to feel guilty about the struggle of the child. Sympathetic one can be, but there ought to be no guilt. Furthermore, such guilt should never be compounded by generating the only handicap that really matters: lack of self-reliance and independence in a society that will only accept reliant and independent members if they are to participate as equals instead of a tolerated fringe.

The burden of meeting that challenge has been given to the schools. They are not often very defensive because they represent the average, but are cajoled by the individuals who feel guilty about the enormity of the task in front of their exceptional child. Yet it is a totally unnecessary approach. Martin McGrath asked:

> Let us feel the bitter as well as the sweet that life usually brings. Let us experience life in its fullness—the sweat, toil and discomfort of leaping over those hurdles of living as well as the joy, pride and warmth that one feels knowing that he has succeeded. Give us the satisfaction of knowing that we have made our markings here on this earth just like everybody else. You may be surprised by what we can become. (2) (p. 51)

To change society is not what the mature handicapped individual wants done for him. They want a chance at changing society themselves. Any attempt to do it for them is spurred by guilt and is, in fact, a most grievous form of rejection. When the exceptional child demands that it be done for him and we comply, we who are unquestioned contributors to the average have failed to handle the problem of the presence of the exceptional. True love is to let go, to allow, to accept as equal, and to listen to aggression without blindly flailing back. Only then does the exceptional child have a chance to become a member of society and to contribute to the average.

REFERENCES

1. Huxley, A. Brave New World. New York: Harper & Row, Publishers, Inc., 1950.
2. McGrath, M. A. Give Us the Knife. Nashville: Ashlan Press, 1978.
3. Kierkegaard, S. The Sickness unto Death. Lowrie, W., translator. Princeton, N.J.: Princeton University Press, 1953.
4. Connor, F. P., Cohen, M., eds. Leadership Preparation for Educators of Crippled and Other Health Impaired-Multiply Handicapped Populations. Report of a Special Study Institute, Tappan Zee Inn, Nyack, N.Y., 1973. New York: Teachers College Press, 1973.
5. van Eys, J. Caring for the child who might die. In: Barton, D., ed. Dying and Death. A Clinical Guide for Caregivers. Baltimore: Williams & Wilkins Co., 1977, pp. 222–236.
6. Goodspeed, B. J. The Apocrypha, An American Translation. Chicago: University of Chicago Press, 1938.
7. John F. Kennedy, Inaugural Address, January 20, 1961. Inaugural Addresses of the Presidents of the United States. House Document 93-208. Washington, D.C.: U.S. Government Printing Office, 1979, pp. 267–270.
8. van Eys, J. The normally sick child. In: van Eys, J., ed. The Normally Sick Child. Baltimore: University Park Press, 1979, pp. 11–27.

CHAPTER 16

The Impact of the Handicapped

ALLISON STOVALL
SUE NICHOLS

Our primary focus in this discussion was on the development of self-acceptance, particularly in those deemed by society to be exceptional. We agreed that differentness is a quality that provides a rich life experience for those of us who choose to work with exceptional children. At the same time, we acknowledged that the individual with an unsound body is often suspected of having an unsound mind by the larger society.

The concept of self-acceptance must be viewed in relation to societal norms. Dr. van Eys defined self-acceptance as accepting where you are in relation to where society is and coming to grips with that. Only after doing so can you decide what to do about society. Attainment of self-acceptance is difficult when we consider the societal norms for performance. It is possible for unrealistic expectations of family and community. When we use our children to confirm our own insecurities, we impede their development of self-acceptance. If parents have to rely on their children's conforming with their belief systems to feel good about themselves, they deny the right of self-acceptance to their children. Social values that reinforce the Protestant ethic of sacrificing for others are interpreted as being mutually exclusive with this concept of self-acceptance.

The movements now in vogue that espouse self-awareness are often counterproductive to the pursuit of self-acceptance. These efforts toward personal growth sometimes place too much emphasis on becoming angry with the self you discover and using that anger to transform that self. Dr. van Eys illustrated this point by referring to the feminist movement. When women discover their capabilities and accept themselves in relationship to their positions in society, then they can engage in the task of changing society. When they look at themselves in relation to men and use their anger to try to become like men, they are moving away from self-acceptance.

When we see this distinction in the uses of self-awareness, we can embrace the positive aspects of self-acceptance. True self-acceptance allows for the expression of anger and of love. As Dr. van Eys said in his presentation, the only way to love is to let go. We illustrated this by examining the disparate concepts of humanity and personhood. Dr. van Eys defined humanity as "being accepted as part of the human herd." In contrast, he said that personhood was "being allowed to act independently in the human herd." There is considerable variation in the timing of the acceptance of personhood, of loving by letting go.

The medically exceptional child's struggle for personhood is complicated by many obstacles. Many people see handicaps as conditions that militate against personhood. We must possess the security to bestow personhood on ourselves as well as having it bestowed upon us. Recognition of one's own personhood is a prerequisite to granting personhood to others. As observers of the caregivers in educational and medical settings, we see that the insecurities that often accompany inexperience inhibit the development of self-acceptance in children. When young people are impatient with their own lives, it is difficult for them to grant personhood to exceptional children. Parents are faced with an ongoing task of enabling their children to attain self-acceptance. Their struggle with this task is more intense than that of nurses, teachers, and physicians. Many find ways to reinforce childhood dependence out of their own guilt and insecurity, particularly with medically exceptional children.

If we who have chosen to work for the optimal development of children can allow them their personhood, we can create for them a world in which exceptionality is not a handicap. The challenge we face is to rid ourselves of the handicap of not accepting ourselves. That accomplished, we can facilitate the process of letting go to love. When that process is successful, children are free to make choices about learning, about living fully within medically imposed limitations, and about dying when they know that it is time for death.

As handicapped persons become more integrated into our day-to-day lives, our perceptions of them change. Our exposure to the handicapped tends to increase our awareness of reality. We see those with special limitations as capable of contributing to society in a positive way. We see ourselves as more accepting of our own limitations as well as those of others. As a result, we may become a more interdependent society, that not only allows but expects each to contribute as well as participate. This change in society is furthered through increased communication, sharing, and a greater awareness of ourselves and others.

CHAPTER 17

Modulating Public Opinion

KATY MAXWELL
BETTY PFEFFERBAUM
DONNA COPELAND
PAUL HANSEN

It is clear from the passage of Public Law 94-142 (Education for All Handicapped Children Act, 1975) that legislators, and presumably the public whom they represent, have some awareness of the special educational needs of exceptional children. The law requires that all children, regardless of handicapping condition, be provided a free, appropriate education, and that the schools make available "related services" (physical therapy, occupational therapy, counseling, social work, and specialized supportive services) to those children who would not otherwise benefit from their educational programs. This brief and general statement may very well reflect the full extent of most people's understanding of the law and its implications. There are many facets of the law that are either unknown or misunderstood by many, and because the law has such broad implications for schools and society, there is a real need to educate the public.

Although many do not realize it, the passage of Public Law 94-142 has dramatically changed the definition of "education." Traditionally, the term has meant "reading, writing, and 'rithmetic'" or "book learning." But the law has mandated that severely and profoundly handicapped children who cannot benefit from traditional education be served by the schools. For these children, the term "education" implicitly refers to anything that will improve the child's quality of life. These children are being taught very basic skills such as grasping objects, chewing food, and toilet training.

In serving such children, the schools' reponsibilities, and thereby the costs, have grown enormously particularly since the law mandates that the most severely handicapped, those children typically needed the most related services met with the least potential for rehabilitation, be given priority for service. Much of the public is unaware that the law dictates the opposite of triage and is unaware of the cost to the taxpayer of serving profoundly handicapped children in public school settings. More fully educating the public to these aspects of the law might result in a change in priorities for tax dollars to benefit the schools. It might even result in a change in the legislation itself.

Public Law 94-142 requires that students be served in the least restrictive envirionment, in that they be mainstreamed as much as is deemed appropriate. The impact of this requirement has been both positive and negative. Many teachers (and parents of regular education students) may feel imposed on when a handicapped student is mainstreamed in a "normal" classroom or when a classroom at a school is used to serve handicapped children. Some educators may feel disconcerted by the reality that teaching encompasses more than traditional activities, but now includes self-help and life-management training. There is a real need for adequate preparation of teachers, parents, and children alike since the law mandates that the "normal" shall come in contact with the "exceptional." Once initial acceptance and understanding are achieved, we may begin to see broader changes in society's attitudes toward the handicapped, since simple exposure to the handicapped may minimize fear and enhance acceptance. Mainstreaming also provides the handicapped with valuable experience in how to cope with a "normal" world.

One effect of the law has been a diffusion of boundaries such that the purviews of the family, the education system, and the health care system are no longer distinct. There is potential long-range benefit to this flexibility. However, the immediate impact has been somewhat overwhelming to all concerned. A major problem is the extensive degree of expectation and responsibility delegated to educators. This has been heightened by the lack of established lines of communication between the educational and medical systems. While a great deal of responsibility has been delegated to the educators, and while the medical profession declares a willingness and ability to participate in total care, the ultimate challenge still rests with the child and his family.

This need for information and public education can be satisfied. Public opinion can be modulated by appropriate modes of communication. Ways in which this can be accomplished include:

> Parents and children visiting schools they are interested in, spending enough time at each place to ask questions and to develop some sense of atmosphere.

> Children are good conveyors of information. Mainstreaming, for example, is a way of educating all children about differences among people, and the exposure to differences is conducive to acceptance. Children will carry this experience outside the classroom.

> Teachers need to be educated in this area as well, and there should be a comprehensive program on the subject included in teacher training. In-service presentations can be helpful, especially if they are proposed in a manner that will appeal to the teachers.

> The medical profession has a role to play in the process, which may be fulfilled a number of ways. First, these professionals can help by preparing families for reintegration, letting them know what to expect, encouraging them to see that their children attend, and informing them of any special considerations their children may require. Second, the medical profession may advise school personnel on any procedures a child may require, or on other matters pertaining to a child's reintegration. Ideally, there would be a

liaison service that would coordinate efforts among the three sectors: hospital, school, and home. And third, it could be proposed that inviting school personnel to the hospital to acquaint them with a child's hospital experience may also be helpful.

Parent organizations may be used to disseminate information. Many of the discussants observed that PTA groups and VIP parents, for example, could be utilized to spread information.

A big problem exists in maintaining the gains we might make. A success may get publicity for a time, but then be ignored later. Today, the media seem more interested in sensationalism than in solid progress. A recent example can be quoted of an older woman who directed a successful pilot project at an elementary school. The news media were more interested in reporting on her motorcycle riding than in her serious work for special children.

Two major conclusions came out of the discussions: Adequately facing the problem and coping with it requires team efforts; the schools, parents, the medical profession, and the media need to be involved in joint efforts to make the general public and people within the professions aware of the task of reintegrating exceptional children. This presupposes the second major point—adequate communication among the differing groups involved, and between these and the community at large. Simple communication is not enough; however, out of these interactions new and useful insights must develop which will ensure that the needs of the children will actually be served, rather than the special interests of small groups and individuals.

Section V

CLOSURE

CHAPTER 18

Cooperation Through Understanding of Needs and Perceptions

JAN VAN EYS

Until very recently, medicine dealt primarily with acute diseases. The miracle of modern medicine was wrought with the understanding of the etiology of acute epidemic diseases. Prevention controlled epidemics and treatment avoided serious sequelae. During that time schools taught well children. A child was either well or too sick to go to school. There was little in between.

Our current medical era is the era of the chronic disease. There is now the recognition that certain variants in physiology and biochemistry in patients are compatible with life with the support of the medical establishment. We cannot yet transplant the pancreas, but the child with diabetes can live a useful life. Childhood cancer is a chronic disease. As a consequence, schools face a problem never foreseen. The methodology to teach the normal child might preclude the exceptional child from learning. Yet, special education helped and hindered at the same time. On the one hand, it managed to teach the exceptional children when the ordinary classroom could not accommodate them. On the other hand, it excluded children from the normal stream of preparation for society. It is from these two, although mutually exclusive, demands for the child that Public Law 94-142 was born.

This process was entirely analogous to the pressure on the medical establishment by the societal forces that demand more than mere biological care for the sick. The phenomenon of holistic medicine is, in principle, born from the demand that care be extended beyond the confines of the setting in which the disease is treated. It is directed to preparation of the patient for a life after or with the disease in ways that are most compatible with productivity and mental health.

In both areas, the school and medicine, these forces created on occasion extremes and, not infrequently, abuses. From the concept of an environment most conducive to learning, we have changed the burden of learning from the student to the teacher. That need not be elaborated. Suffice it to say that one cannot teach complex concepts when the pupil has but few words.

The extremes in medicine are just as evident. We went from the supportive and descriptive analysis of the process of dying of Kübler-Ross (1) to the unfounded theosophy of reincarnation of the dead (2), endorsed by the same psychiatrist. We went from maximizing inner resources to centers for attitudinal healing (3), with all the burdens of guilt that one can heap on unsuspecting children: when they become convinced, they can overcome their cancer by mind set.

But we must never lose sight of a correct principle just because, in practice, it is frequently misinterpreted. To have a chronic disease is a state of life. Therefore, medical attention is never enough. Furthermore, the physicians are rarely the persons best suited to help the sick beyond their physical needs. Yet, to be in school with a chronic illness creates problems well beyond those of special education skills.

Schooling is one of the primary tasks of the child—ill or well. A child has numerous interactions and learning challenges during the day. However, for the medically exceptional children with their life distorted from what one would have hoped, the major elements in shaping life are family, education, and medical care. In other words, if there were an equal partnership between parents and child with medical care and education, the charge of total care for the chronically ill child would be met to a very large degree through cooperation between medical personnel and educators. Similarly, the challenges of Public Law 94-142 would be greatly helped when these professionals cooperate in designing meaningful supplementations for that law's mandates. To make the exceptional child maximally functional there is a responsibility for physicians to identify the medically exceptional child, to evaluate the child, and to continue the provision of medical services to optimize the potential of participation in school (4,5). Yet, there is precious little in the educational literature describing this interaction in a constructive way. A review by Guralnick et al. of the literature of special education failed to reveal any descriptive or investigative articles on existing collaborative efforts between pediatricians and special educators (6). It is clear that our current side by side efforts, without collaboration, are not just wasted, but are, in fact, counterproductive. The duplication of services, evaluations, reviews, and conferences can be enormous. Even if both school and medical personnel talk with each other, there is no guarantee that there is a dialogue, and even when there is a dialogue, that there is mutual instruction and support.

This phenomenon of side-by-side teamwork without true cooperation is rampant in the world of complex care delivery. As a typical example in the area of total medical care, the case of a mother of a child with rubella syndrome can be cited (7). The medical establishment saw to it that this 3½-year-old child received total care. He had congenital cataracts, congenital heart disease, a hemolytic anemia, a transient platelet deficiency, slow motor and mental development, deafness, and feeding problems. He was receiving services from the following agencies: The Baltimore City Health Department through their Well Baby Clinic and Division for the Handicapped; The Maryland State Department of Health through the Crippled Children's Services and Community Services to the Mentally Retarded; The Johns Hopkins Hospital in the Cardiac Clinic, Speech and Hearing Center, Child Growth and Development Study, the Eye Clinic, the Pediatric Clinic, and the Emergency Room; The Greater Baltimore Medical Center in their Comprehensive Pediatric Clinic; The Children's Hospital Orthopedic Clinic; The Hearing and Speech Agency of Metropolitan Baltimore, by enrollment in the Gateway Preschool; The School for the Blind, in preparation for admission; Tentative evaluation for day-care services for the mentally retarded; and tentative evaluation for Rosewood State Hospital (7). The mother was so burdened with the total care of her child that she could do nothing else. Nor could the child really profit from the services, since he was so busy being helped that he could not develop.

The need is defined by the goal of both education and medical care for the exceptional child: the realization of the maximum performance of which the child is capable for the total life span. That means realistic appraisal of potential; therefore, it also means to be objective. It does not leave room for the championing of a personal opinion. It does not allow the manipulation of a system to make a personal point. The quality of life is determined by the child, not the teacher or the doctor. The child has the potential. The professionals who are asked to help must assist to realize such potential as is found in that specific child. There are no generalizations in approach. The generalization lies in the goal, the body of knowledge, and the resources and skills the child needs.

There is much we do not know about the socialization of the medically exceptional child. The cooperation between school and medicine must contain the three elements necessary in any endeavor that is not totally stylized and fixed: care, research, and education.

Care ought to be a collaborative undertaking. There should be a demonstration project in which the care for a child is jointly planned by educators and medical personnel. The educational method for generalizing individualized progress is the ARD Conference—Admission, Review and Dismissal, in which parents, educators, and information support personnel match the capabilities of the child to the available educational environment in order that the goals set by the parents can be met to the greatest possible degree. Having thereby set educational objectives, the primary teacher can write an IEP, an Individualized Education Plan. The medical community utilizes a staffing conference in which all elements of the care delivery for the child report their observations and objectives to generate a cohesive program that maximally supports the realistic medical objective, be that total care or palliative support. The teachers have in their ARD a token medical report, and the physicians, nurses, and mental health workers have in their staffing a token teacher. Both are often more concerned about the mechanics of the establishment than with the reality of the child's world.

A care project in which a combined total program is generated through a combined complete ARD would demonstrate the feasibility of truly integrated care. The time required to do this for all chronically ill children would be prohibitive, or if sufficient professional personnel could be found, the cost would still be prohibitively expensive. But from a well-described demonstration program where this principle is put into action, guidelines could be generated that could be used to develop a basic plan of approach for all children. Currently there is no common language, let alone a common manual, that can be understood by medical and educational personnel.

Continuing education of the involved professional is the long-range solution. All personnel must be aware of the problems inherent in the setting of the other group. There are new suggestions for curricula development for pediatric trainees to understand the world of the handicapped (8). But those proposals still do not fully appreciate the concepts that are used in the schools for teaching and guidance in development. A chronically ill child is a patient under active care only a few hours a month and a pupil several hours a day.

Not infrequently do the parents use the physicians as unsuspecting allies in their private demands for a special consideration from the schools. Physicians unthinkingly certify homebound teaching when there is really no justification, except that parents want it. Conversely, children are certified to be in need of expensive medical facilities that are certified as necessary to pursue an education. The school system is, thereby, financially burdened with what ought to be medical costs and not educational costs.

Both educators and medical care personnel ought to strive for the goal of a "truly cured child" (9). Both must consider the chronically ill child a normally sick child (10). It is normal for a child to be sick and a sick child is normal. To deal with that reality, these professionals must develop a common voice about the goals for the child. It is the medically exceptional children who must feel good about themselves. Only that will make the goal of a normally reintegrated child a reality (11). The teaching must be directed at the medical and educational establishments so that the parents can be taught about the reality of an environment conducive to teaching the children to feel good about themselves. It is a three-step process.

There is much we do not know about the child who is medically handicapped. The problems surrounding the approach to the extreme physical handicap is that most deal with the physical obstacles that common society places in the way of the handicapped. However, the challenge lies in optimal self-development. The generation of a good self-image is indeed mixed with generating opportunities for accomplishment. However, that is a means toward an end.

The problem presented by cancer in children is a clear example of the separativeness of the problem. The life-threatening nature of childhood cancer, the chronicity of the treatment, and the potential long-range after-effects of therapy (12) all generate a real, tangible handicap. But the real handicap is the child's self-image and the reaction of society to the perceived potential in the child. It is especially in this disease that the research can be most fruitfully conducted because the two elements, physical and mental, are so readily separated. However, only now are data emerging.

It must be remembered that such data are a process. Medicine moves rapidly. Again when we look up the impact of a given method of therapy, a specific late effect on the development of self-image, we miss the point. No doubt an amputation for osteosarcoma is a threatening experience. An attempt at limb salvage for that disorder will change the mental outlook and challenge for the child. But the method by which we might help make the child cope is similar. The facts are real and they incorporate a most significant change for the child. We would not substitute our belief about being able to offer less mutilative approaches for our empathy with the ego-shattering experience that being totally helpless brings. It is not really so difficult to assimilate what is being done, as it is that it is being done.

Research must direct itself at understanding the basic drives of children. It must be an investigation of ontology. That is very basic research in this area. Therefore, it cannot be executed except by a very few. However, we should listen to those researchers, be they psychologists, theologians, or historians. Using their clues we should design our environment such that we capitalize on the natural drive to grow and develop. Children are basically geared to developing normally. That does not mean they develop uniformly. But our environment must allow the development of potential. That does not mean simply adapting the hospital and classrooms so that the handicapped do not encounter unnecessary obstacles. That ought not ever be an issue. You cannot teach the blind with pictures or the deaf with records and audiotapes. It ought to be self-evident that the means are adaptive for the target to reach a goal. It is the goal that must be uniform as defined.

In medicine the concept is the therapeutic community. The environment is part of the therapy and should be responsive to the total needs of the child. In education there should be no less. The school building itself, just as the hospital, should represent the concept of the desired goal. How that can best be realized is the subject of needed research. Not detailed research, which assumes the transient as the fixed, but research as self-development while a child with a chronic illness has special needs, basically, it is still a child, only more so. We must deal with them with anticipating guidance (13).

The impact of medically exceptionality is enormous. In school age it is approximately one percent of all children. If you add mild variants such as partial hearing loss or moderate physical impairment, the figure may rise staggeringly. Fifty out of 1000 school children have abnormal hearing levels in one or both ears, with half of those potentially affected by that defect, while 5 out of 1000 are overtly hard of hearing (14). Even more surprising are the figures for children with cancer. While cancer in children is a rare disease, in the course of their childhood 1 in 600 children will contract cancer. That extrapolates to an attack rate of 1 in 9000 to 1 in 10,000 per year. Now that we cure up to 60% the incidence of cured cancer in the population will soon be 1 in 1000 (15). That is a veritable epidemic of maladjustment if we allow the mental health of such individuals to be a secondary concern, if we make it a concern at all.

Medicine must surely change to accept variance in health as being normal. Deviations in self-acceptance must become the target of concern. Since we do not do this yet, the phrase of Doctor Knowles, President of the Rockefeller Foundation, does apply: "Doing better and feeling worse" (16).

There must be a concerted effort in shifting the balance between accepting oneself as one really is and being defeatist about what one could become. Again, cancer gives the best example. The disease is almost invariably fatal when not treated. We now can cure at a price. To decide that the price is not worth it can only be done by the patients themselves. But once the price is decided upon, once the risk is taken, there ought not to be any guilt about having exacted the price.

There must be cooperation between professionals in medicine and education. They ought to have the same goal. They ought not to have unrealistic expectations of each other. They should agree first on the physical and immediate needs of the handicapped, so that generating the ability to have good quality of life becomes possible. Then they ought to go on with the business at hand, teaching children to realize their potential by motivating them, teaching them self-acceptance, and making self-reliance possible. That is not a problem in mechanical barriers, but a problem in perception.

REFERENCES

1. Kübler-Ross, E. Death and Dying. New York: Macmillan, Inc., 1969.
2. Head, J., Cranston, S. L. Reincarnation: The Phoenix Mystery. New York: Crown Publishers, Inc., 1972.
3. Jampolsky, G., Taylor, P. Foreword. In: There Is a Rainbow behind Every Dark Cloud. Millbrae, Calif.: Celestial Arts, 1978.
4. Jacobs, M. J., Walker, D. K. Pediatrics and the education for all handicapped children. Act of 1975 (Public Law 94-142). Pediatrics, 61:135–137, 1978.
5. Palfrey, J. D., Mervis, R. C., Butler, J. A. New directions in the evaluation and education of handicapped children. N. Engl. J. Med., 298:819–824, 1978.
6. Guralnick, M. J., Richardson, M. B., Jr., Kutner, D. R. Pediatric education and the development of exceptional children. In: Guralnick, M. J., Richardson, M. B., Jr., eds. Pediatric Education and the Needs of Exceptional Children. Baltimore: University Park Press, 1980, pp. 3–19.
7. Hopkins, E. The chronically ill child and the community. In: Debussey, M., ed. The Chronically Ill Child and His Family. Springfield, Ill.: Charles C Thomas, Publisher, 1970, pp. 196–198.
8. Richardson, M. B., Jr., Guralnick, M. J., Taft, L. T., Levine, M. D. A comprehensive curriculum in child development and handicapping conditions. Prospect for design, implementation, and evaluation. In: Guralnick, M. J., Richardson, M. B., Jr., eds. Pediatric Education and the Needs of Exceptional Children. Baltimore: University Park Press, 1980, pp. 185–202.
9. van Eys, J., ed. The Truly Cured Child. Baltimore: University Park Press, 1978.
10. van Eys, J. The normally sick child. In: van Eys, J., ed. The Normally Sick Child. Baltimore: University Park Press, 1979, pp. 11–27.

11. van Eys, J. Changing society is not the best solution. Proceedings of the Fifth Annual Mental Health Conference, Reintegration of the Medically Exceptional child, Houston, Texas, April 25–26, 1980. These Proceedings pp. 129–150.
12. Jaffe, J., O'Malley, J. E., Koocher, G., Foster, D., Gogan, J., Li, F. P., Fine, W. The cost of therapy. In: van Eys, J., ed. The Normally Sick Child. Baltimore: University Park Press, 1979, pp. 67–79.
13. Brazelton, T. B. Anticipatory guidance. Pediatr. Clin. North Am., 22: 533–544, 1975.
14. Eagles, E. L., Wishik, S. M., Deurfler, L., Melnick, W., Levine, M. S. Hearing sensitivity and related factors in children. (NINDH grant NB-02375-074) Laryngoscope June 1973.
15. Meadows, A. T., Krejmas, N., Belasco, J. For the Late Effects Study Group. The medical cost of cure: Sequelae in survivors of childhood cancer. In: van Eys, J., Sullivan, M. P., eds. Status of the Curability of Childhood Cancers. New York: Raven Press, 1980, pp. 263–275.
16. Knowles, J. M., ed. Doing Better and Feeling Worse. Health in the United States. New York: W. W. Norton & Co., Inc., 1977.

CHAPTER 19

Closure

PATRICIA SHELL

Our topic has been the reintegration of the medically excep-tional child. During this conference, we talked with one another and we thought individually a great deal about all aspects of this topic. In doing so, we have dealt with the role, including the rights and responsibilities, of the family, medicine, and education. We have explored the ethical and philosophical issues of reintegration. We have talked about the financial issues and legal ramifications involved. Indeed, we have said in several ways that we would not have held a conference like this in 1959 or the early 1960s. We have reflected that a growing awareness of the needs of these children was really put into a legal framework in the late 1960s and the 1970s.

We talked about the political issues and ramifications brought to bear on the medical and educational communities, and indeed on the family. Even the family dynamics may themselves be thought of as one manifestation of the operation of political issues.

And throughout it all, we dealt with the human issues involved. I think it is that thread that I have seen underlying what has been expressed by each speaker, whether that speaker represented the medical community, the educational community, or the family and home. Many times throughout this conference as I have listened, I have seen the three spheres: hospital, home, and school. But the one variable common to all is the medically exceptional child. It is this child who moves into and out of that home, that hospital, and that school. It is this child who becomes the focus in varying ways at various times in his life. Even throughout a single day he moves into and out of, between and among, those spheres that form the setting that is his world.

As we talk about the reintegration of the medically exceptional child, reintegration from a focus solely in the world of medicine to that outside the world of medicine, we have to think about the school, that part of the child's life primarily outside the home. So it was with extreme pleasure that we in the Houston Independent School District responded to the invitation to join with The University of Texas System Cancer Center in this conference. We too have felt and continue to feel very sharply the need for this kind of interchange. We feel this not only in our own school district, but in school districts throughout the state and the nation with whom we have ongoing communication concerning the education of handicapped children. We feel that we have become much better collectors of information about children than we once were. The mere size of the stacks of paper attests that we at least collect more pieces of paper with more kinds of reports speaking to the intellectual functioning of the child and his performance of various educational tasks within the school setting. We concur that many times the information we have about the child's physical being, including the state of his health, is extremely sketchy, often not understood by us even if we have very complete information. And we already suspected what the medical community confirmed during this conference, that many times the medical team has not had the information for that part of the child's world that does indeed occupy a large portion of his thinking, his time, and his whole being, the school.

We realize that Public Law 94-142 was addressed to educators. It was specifically addressed to the school. It lays very specific and very cumbersome mandates on the public education system in this country. It is unfortunate that the law was not phrased in such a way that it was evident early on that it also affects the medical community. While it was addressed to the public schools, because the mandate for its implementation rests with the public schools, it is also addressed to the medical community and to parents.

We have said that the home, the hospital, and the school need somehow to be blended so that the circles interlock. They must not remain three isolated spheres if we are to serve the child appropriately, and if the child is to be given the opportunity to assert her own responsibility for her reactions to herself and to the world about her. Somehow our mission must be to bring about an interlocking of those circles so that they do indeed mirror where we touch the child.

This conference is one step towards doing that. But what have we accomplished here? We came thinking that we were going to find answers to specific questions, and we probably now have some new questions. In fact, I would hope that each of us has new questions to ask. At the very bottom level, surely for each of us who have participated in the conference and for those who will read the proceedings, there will be a raised level of awareness of the score, of the problem, of what the issue really is. I hope there will be a sense of commitment to being a part of making things different and better for the medically exceptional child. Optimally, I would hope that this conference is one more bridge into a kind of communication that involves the home, school, and the medical community in a dialogue that sees a merging of our operations and implementations of our own programs, our own goals in such a way that the medically exceptional child does benefit by being reintegrated into the whole of society with all of us working with her.

We appreciate as a school district the opportunity for our teachers, our special education support personnel, our principals, and our central office administrators, to be a part of this conference and we hope that it is but the first step in an ongoing effort.

CHAPTER 20

Postscript — Perspectives of the Convener

DONNA R. COPELAND

The Conference on the Reintegration of the Medically Exceptional Child was conceived by people who are dedicated to the welfare and guidance of all children and who particularly recognize that some children have special needs. The conference was a success, judging from the enthusiasm, spirit of collaboration, expertise, and experience. And underlying these exceptional qualities was a keen awareness of the problems associated with educating medically exceptional children; but along with it too were optimism and determination to seek solutions and make change a reality.

As noted by a number of speakers, the task was defined by virtue of the success in cancer treatment for children during the last few years. But surviving cancer is an achievement won at significant cost, for it often includes, among other consequences, setbacks in the educational experience—hence in socialization and development, in other words, a lack of normalcy. The conference participants were aware that this interruption need not be permanent; it only means that this extra effort is required by more people to achieve reintegration in its finest sense.

The conference was part of a series of conferences that began five years ago, the sequence of which reflects not only the progress in cancer treatment for children, but also our views toward chronic illness. First, we considered the concept of cure and what that means for the parties involved (1), along with the implications of research on children during treatment (2). Then we recognized the importance of accepting the child's illness as normal (3) and tried to sort through the multitude of experiences and feelings cancer evokes in the child, the parents, and those who administer the care (4). It was timely then, after these considerations, to turn toward the school as a setting where much of the child's normalcy is defined—a place where the child can be "truly cured" (1).

The conference brought together three basic disciplines—medicine, education, and mental health—in a joint effort to understand better one another's perspective and thus approach the task of integration more rationally and more realistically, that is, from a viewpoint closer to what the child actually sees. Simply being together, listening to one another, and becoming better acquainted with one another and with each person's perspectives and tasks was beneficial in itself. Awareness is the first order of business in any meaningful approach toward a goal, and seeing other views broadens the scope of one's own. But beyond this, significant steps were made toward establishing a foundation upon which a viable communication, planning, and liaison service could perhaps one day be built.

There were formal and informal segments of the conference to help us view the problems in historical and present contexts and to help us integrate our thinking about what might be done. It was necessary and helpful, as well as inspiring, to listen to the formal presentations on legal, educational, psychosocial, and medical backgrounds contributing to the current status of handicapped children. Then, to build upon these, and in keeping with the philosophy of the benefits of active involvement of participants, wo noodod to talk with ono anothor, dovolop rapport, and sharo experiences and ideas thus enriching the conference and providing the opportunity for the crucial first steps in collaboration.

The commitment of the participants was obvious to me, but along with it, balancing the enthusiasm and optimism, was a healthy dose of skepticism. A plea for realistic goals was heard as well. We were reminded that the concept of rehabilitating the handicapped is relatively new to our society and to some extent conflicts with some commonly held attitudes about their "help-lessness." We were reminded of the limitations of what is possible for us to achieve (living in an imperfect world) and we disagreed on how far the parameters of our responsibility should extend.

Acceptance of the reality of an imperfect world helps in defining our goals: rather than working for a perfect world, an impossible task, we can teach children how to deal with the frustration and prejudice they will encounter and to take risks that will strengthen and move them further along in growth and self-fulfillment.

Yes, we do have idealism, but with uncertainties—uncertainties about how best to provide for children and to do it equitably; uncertainties about what to expect from parents, the schools, the medical community, and the child; uncertainties about whether our good intentions will achieve the perfection toward which we strive; uncertainties about the disappointment that follows anything short of full accomplishment.

But this is healthy. Skepticism and doubt have a way of keeping us honest and staying on task, while idealism serves to create promising hopes and new possibilities.

Our successes, and failures, will be relative, gauged by each one's individual experience and the measures we learned to use in childhood.

> Every adult whether he is a follower or a leader, a member of a mass or of an elite, was once a child. He was once small. A sense of smallness forms a substratum in his mind, ineradicably. His triumphs will be measured against this smallness, his defeats will substantiate it. (5)

Our task is set: The smallness in the child—and in the child in us—must eventually be rendered insignificant, as dependency is transformed into dependability and independent living, and as we become more confident that we and others do make a difference, that we can be effective in endeavors such as these which we choose to undertake.

REFERENCES

1. van Eys, J., ed. The Truly Cured Child. Baltimore: University Park Press, 1977.
2. van Eys, J., ed. Research on Children. Baltimore: University Park Press, 1978.
3. van Eys, J., ed. The Normally Sick Child. Baltimore: University Park Press, 1970.
4. van Eys, J., ed. Experiencing cancer care: Lore and science. Cancer Bulletin, 32:3–36, 1980.
5. Erikson, E. H. Childhood and Society. New York: W. W. Norton and Co., 1963, p. 404.

Index